Online Survey

Merlin Waltz

Most of this story is 100% true. It's based on actual events. Some statements are based on opinion and I've added to it in order to make it entertaining. There is some information which would be considered hearsay in a court of law, and in those cases, I've done my best to clarify and make the reader aware of it. Some statements are based on the unknown and I've done my best to clarify that information as well. When one is going public with a story that has global "Whistleblower" overtones attached, one must be careful and tread lightly. Too bad I'm not the type to be overly careful or tread lightly, but in this case I've tried to practice a little restraint. Any resemblance to any real or actual events, places, or people, living or dead, is not coincidental, but possibly intentional, in some cases. Names, characters, organizations, places, events, descriptions and portrayals, are products of the imagination and experience of the author. The names were changed to protect the guilty and the innocent.

Here are some of my favorite quotes to help set the tone for this story:

"It's better to live one day as a lion than a thousand years as a lamb." Jimmy Page

"I'd rather be hated for who I am than loved for who I am not." Kurt Cobain

"The truth will come to light." William Shakespeare

"When fortune smiles on something as violent and ugly as revenge, it seems proof like no other that not only does God exist, you're doing his will." The Bride - from the movie Kill Bill

Table of Contents

Chapter 1

"Revenge is a dish best served properly."

There was an engineer who worked for Morton Thiokol. He was an honest man. Many have never heard of him. On the evening before the launch of the Challenger space shuttle, he was the engineer who told everyone they should not launch the shuttle due to the cold temperature. He had evidence which showed enough reasonable doubt to abort the launch. The management at Morton Thiokol didn't agree with his concerns, neither did the management from NASA. They didn't err on the side of caution. They didn't care that they were risking lives if they chose to launch. In my opinion, the managers from NASA and Morton Thiokol who were involved in the decision to launch should have all been charged with murder.

The next morning, NASA wanted a signed release from Morton Thiokol prior to the shuttle launch. This engineer was the engineer on-site. He refused to sign it. He told NASA he didn't feel it was safe to launch. NASA was furious and contacted Morton Thiokol and obtained a fax with a signed authorization from an upper manager at Morton Thiokol. They proceeded with the launch. We all know what happened next. The shuttle exploded and seven human lives were lost.

At the hearings, held by the Rogers Commission, this man came forward and told the commission he recommended not launching, but was ignored by the management at NASA and Morton Thiokol. He told the truth.

The following Monday, when he reported to his office, he was told he would no longer be working in the Engineering department. He was told to report to the scheduling department. This was retribution for his honesty. Morton Thiokol was angry because he was honest and wouldn't lie for them, nor would he hide the truth of what really took place prior to launch.

The story you are about to read is also based on the truth. The truth was told by multiple employees at a company where I once worked, but management didn't care. This story is based on my experience. I began writing this story in the year 2016 after learning one of my predictions came true. These events happened during a nine year period prior to 2010. There are many who will not be happy about the information being shared in this story. There are some who will say I should have tried a different approach to resolving the issues and problems shared in this story.

Multiple conspiracies took place at this company and I feel it would have done no good in the long run. I'm using the word conspiracy in one of it's broader interpretations. I don't want to lead anyone to believe it was a criminal conspiracy, but I believe there might have been some crimes committed. In my opinion, there were some felonies committed. I believe some people will agree with the previous statements.

I need to make it clear I'm not the only person who was affected by the actions (or inactions) taken by various members of the management team I worked under. Multiple employees were treated unfairly and had retribution taken against them due to being honest on an Online Survey. Some employees may not have realized what really happened. Some may tell you they were also aware of these facts, but felt nobody in the company really cared. Retribution was taken against multiple employees because we were honest and management couldn't handle it. When a conspiracy takes place, it's nearly impossible to know where to turn. I, like a few others, chose to leave. I chose to bite my tongue, knowing the day would come when some of these events would be made public. I feel I've been inspired and destined to write this story. No, a burning bush did not tell me to do it. Since becoming a writer and an amateur reporter, I was inspired by a burning desire to expose and share these experiences.

This book won't read like the typical story. It won't read like the typical book. There's a reason for that. I'm saving some juice for the screenplay. I'm doing this intentionally. I'm doing it on purpose. I'm doing what is known as reverse-marketing. When the movie comes out, it will not be verbatim per the book. It will have more in it and it will be different. Why will there be more? Why will it be different? Now that the truth is coming out, I suspect multiple people will be contacting me and sharing their personal experiences with some of the tactics I'm exposing here. It's my hope that they do just that. It's part of my master plan. I want to make it perfectly clear I will protect the privacy of anyone who wants to share information with me. I will revise this book and add their input, if they desire it, or I will use it only in the movie. I'll be very open-minded and do what you feel is best. But know this: the movie will be made. I've already started working on the script. I know this book will be made into a movie. How do I know? Because it's based on the truth.

The company I'm referring to has failed in my opinion. It was taken over by another company in the year 2016. Now, I'm going public and saying: "I told you so." This story will show you some of the reasons why they failed, in my opinion. I knew in my heart, mind, body, and soul this company was destined to fail. It was their own fault. This story will show multiple examples which contributed to their failure. Multiple former co-workers of mine might remember I once said: "If the entire company is being run the way this department is being run, they're going to end up bankrupt." Although they didn't actually go bankrupt, to my knowledge, it's my opinion they failed and were forced to allow the company to be absorbed by another. I'm reminded of an old saying: You can't save your face and your tail at the same time.

The events I'll describe took place in a hospital. I need to make one thing perfectly clear: At no time was there a direct impact to patient care. No patient was ever denied the best possible care. This company always took pride in putting patient care at the top of the list. I would go there for treatment today, if needed. Since patient care wasn't directly impacted, why does it matter? This story will explain why it matters. Later in the story, you will learn of the indirect impact it has. When companies are run in this way, it's my opinion their leadership lives with the delusion everything's fine. They wouldn't even consider multiple employees with over five or ten years of service left their company due to a management problem. With all the courage, strength, and conviction I can muster, I'm here to tell you there was a very serious management problem.

I once stated the entire company was heading for trouble if somebody didn't wake up and smell the coffee or start smelling what they were really shoveling. Now, years later, I have the unhappy honor of saying: I told you so. I said it for years, but it fell on deaf ears. There are those who will say this company did not fail, but chose to pursue an alliance which would better serve the healthcare needs of the community in which it resides. It's my opinion they were heading for failure and there weren't very many ways to avoid it without major changes to the way they were doing business. One example might be the amount they give back to the community. It's my opinion if they continued on of their own accord, they would have had to make drastic changes and cuts in order to stay sufficiently solvent.

Why did I write this story? I wrote this story to let others know they're not alone. I know things like this happen on a regular basis all over this great nation and I think it's a terrible shame. I want the person who has been in similar situations to know someone cares. I care. I feel for you. I know what it feels like because I've been there. I know the amount of anxiety and depression which can overwhelm you when things like this happen. I know there are many who suffer from PTSD due to things like this happening in the workplace. I won't tell you about the major depression I suffered, the anger I had, or the guilt I carried for years over this mess. And all because I cared and because I was honest. The more you care, the more it hurts when you go through things like this. I feel for you. I've been in your shoes. Maybe you've been in my shoes.

Either way, it's a shame things like this are still going on in the twenty-first century of our existence. You give 200% and you get lies, lip-service, and bull-squat in return. You give 200% and you're given the honor of watching someone get hired off the street in a high-paying position you were told you couldn't even apply for. And in some cases, there's not a darn thing you can do about it. I know there are some who have turned to violence when things like this happen. Luckily, I've never been the violent type, but I can surely see how a person could come to the conclusion violence is their only resolve. I'm not saying I agree to violence being used as a resolution. I'm stating when a person is pushed too far, anything is possible and all bets are off.

You sometimes hear about those who chose violence as their resolution to a workplace problem. The media usually says it was a "disgruntled employee." The media won't usually get the rest of the story. They won't dig deep enough to find out what really happened. In other words: Was the employee justifiably disgruntled? Did certain things happen to cause said employee to resort to violence? Or did said employee just wake up one morning and decide to go shoot up the workplace?

I'm not a disgruntled employee. What happened to me begins with a "dis" but the word is not disgruntled. The word is: Discrimination. I'm an employee who was discriminated against on more than one occasion. I was discriminated against multiple ways and multiple times. You'll learn more about it later in the story. Has the media ever started a story with the phrase: "An employee who was discriminated against by Company X came in and shot up the place today. Many shared they were surprised he didn't do it sooner. Some shared the management were scum and treated multiple employees very poorly." Isn't it surprising in 240 years of existence our nation has never had a newspaper story with such a headline? I wonder why? Are you going to tell me it was never the case? If so, I personally would find it very hard to believe.

There are a few other reasons I wrote this story. I'm flushing out a few rats. To flush out a rat, you need some really good bait. I think this story will do the trick. I'm also going to find out if the CEO is a man of honor and integrity. If he is, then maybe he'll put some rats out on the street. If I were a CEO and found out various managers in my company made a bold-faced liar out of me, I would definitely put them out on the street. It wouldn't matter if it were ten years later or twenty years later. Do I believe this CEO is a bold-faced liar? No. In my heart of hearts I find it very hard to believe. I would have an easier time believing multiple managers made a bold-faced liar out of him, without his knowledge. I do hold the CEO partially responsible and you will read about the reasons later on. After you read this story, you might agree. One thing's for sure: Now that some of the truth is coming out, more of the truth will come out. It might not all come out, but I feel a good bit of it will. I know the previous statement doesn't make a lot of sense, but if you've ever had to flush out a rat, it would make perfect sense. Another reason for this story is I want to find out about these new so-called "Allies" or "Partners" who recently got involved with this hospital. I'd like to see how they respond to this. I wonder if they'll keep the rat, or rats, and say something like: "Well, it didn't happen while they were in our employ, so no-harm, no-foul." But in reality, I think everyone involved in this fiasco will probably say: "No comment."

Who did I write this story for? I wrote this story to let a certain CEO know I, and others deserved much better. I want this CEO to know he exists in a world of delusion if he thinks all of his managers and senior managers are the great leaders they pretend to be. I want him to know a few of them deserve to be out on the street. Some will consider this harsh and very unprofessional. Keep that in mind when you get to the end of the story. You may change your mind by the time you get to the end of this story.

Who would possibly have any interest in hearing such a story? Anyone who likes hearing about the little guy getting a break or the underdog finally coming out on top. I doubt I'll come out on top when all is said and done, but the satisfaction I now have is priceless. Nobody would, or could, ever understand how good I feel at this moment, unless they walked a mile in my shoes.

If you are a CEO anywhere in this country, you might want to read this story. This story will show you what not to do. This story will suggest changes you may need to make. This story will show you how to avoid having a loose canon like me write a book about you or your company some day. It will also show what can happen when you don't listen to your Microsoft Certified Professional's advice.

There's one downside about a story of this nature: It will give certain types of leaders ideas about how to screw people over and still look good on paper. It will show you how to setup a conspiracy and take retribution against employees you don't like. I hate to give certain types of people the ammunition to do these things, but there's no way to tell this story without showing all sides of the events which took place where I once worked.

Chapter 2

I'm staring at the Sunday paper. I've just made the front page. The headline reads: "Hospital employee to host seminar in Las Vegas. Merlin Waltz, an employee in the IT Department at our local hospital will be hosting a seminar about specialized healthcare software deployments. It will be a kickoff to a newly created position: Software Deployment Specialist. In this newly created role, Merlin will continue addressing local software deployment, which has saved the company over half a million dollars in direct labor costs during the five-plus years he's been engaged in these deployments. He will also be doing consulting work to assist other hospitals nationwide with the implementation and necessary training to perform these customized deployments. This will be a win-win for the hospital, who has achieved great success in the past with sub-contracting IT services to other healthcare facilities. The hospital predicts over a half-million in yearly revenue for this specialized consulting work and this revenue is the result of one person's labor. The biggest news is that 75% of this revenue is total profit, even after overhead and expenses. This is huge by healthcare standards. Aside from physicians, no individual non-clinical employee creates this much revenue and profit for the company or saves the company this much in direct labor fees on a regular basis."

"This solidifies what I've always said about our success being dependent upon recruiting and retaining the best people and treating them well. This is a perfect example. Having managers who recognize and properly reward true talent is one of our greatest assets. In this company, I make it a point of stressing the importance of properly looking for and rewarding true talent and finding previously undiscovered revenue streams," the CEO was quoted as saying.

I wish I could tell you this was how the story ended, but sadly, it isn't the case. It could have been the case and it should have been the case, but it wasn't the case.

I'm staring at the Sunday paper. The headline reads: "Trouble along the Susquehanna." The CEO of our local hospital just issued this press release: "I've terminated a Vice President, two Directors and two Managers from within our IT Department due to a conspiracy which took place. It came to my attention they attempted to corrupt the Online Survey process and were taking retribution against various employees for answering the survey questions honestly and giving negative feedback. This will not be tolerated. The award for 'Best State Employer' is linked to these questions. For that process to be corrupted, it would mean we aren't a 'Best State Employer.' Therefore, I fired them. I'm going public to prove I'm a CEO of honor and integrity who will not allow this company's good name to be tarnished and won't shove things under the carpet. I'm also sending a message to all managers in this company: You mess with the survey, you mess with your future. I'm also letting everyone know the issues and concerns of the employees of the IT Department are now being properly addressed, and the new management team understands the importance of it."

I wish I could tell you this was how the story ended, but that's not the case. It could have been the case and it should have been the case, but it wasn't the case.

Chapter 3

The courtroom is no different than any other courtroom. The walls are covered with a fine wood finish. The bench has a short flag pole on each side. There's an American flag on the left and the Pennsylvania state flag on the right. It's not a huge courtroom. It's about the size one would expect to find in an area with a population of one hundred thousand. The courtroom is empty today, with the exception of a bailiff standing beside the door leading to the judges chambers. There's one person sitting on a bench in the hallway outside the courtroom. His name is Randy Chester. He's a former employee of the IT Department at Riverside Health System. He just arrived a few minutes ago and sent Merlin a text announcing his arrival.

The jury selection process is supposed to begin tomorrow. A pre-trial meeting is currently being held in the judges chambers. Pre-trial meetings are quite common. Various motions are made and decisions about admissible evidence is being discussed. This pre-trial meeting is going to be a little different. The plaintiff is representing himself. The defense attorney for Riverside Health System, Boris Angelino, is present. William Hocks, the CEO of Riverside Health System is also present. There is also a stenographer present. The honorable James Hinson is the first to speak.

"Mr. Waltz, You need to understand the request you are making should have come much sooner.

We're supposed to begin the jury selection process tomorrow. This is a very serious accusation. It should have been made before the discovery process began. Why did you wait until now to come forward with this motion?" Asks Judge Hinson.

"I'm sorry your honor. I wasn't able to locate the witness until yesterday," replied Merlin Waltz, the plaintiff.

"Was there a subpoena issued for this witness?" Asked Judge Hinson.

"No, your honor. There was not. I wanted this witness to come forward with no coercion," replied Merlin.

"Mr. Waltz, I've given you a lot of latitude, due to the fact you've chosen to represent yourself. I've suggested you find an attorney to assist you with this case. A competent attorney would have made this request much sooner. I'm going to share your motion with the defense. I'm also going to hear from your witness. I will then make a decision based on the testimony."

"Thank-You, your honor. I apologize for my inexperience. If the defendants will allow it, I will seek a competent legal attorney to assist me with the remainder of the trial. But only if the defendants agree to it. If they don't agree to it, I will have no choice but to continue representing myself," replied Merlin.

Mr. Angelino and the CEO were whispering to each other. The judge waited patiently until they were done with their private conversation.

"Mr. Angelino? Would you like to respond to the statement just made by the plaintiff?" Asks the judge.

"We have no objection to Mr. Waltz obtaining legal representation. He has the right to change his mind. He has the right to be properly represented. If we were to deny him this request, he would have grounds for a mistrial. We surely don't want that to happen and we surely don't want to delay these proceedings any longer," replied the defense attorney.

Merlin is keeping a straight face. He's saying nothing. He's wearing his poker face. He's laughing his tail off on the inside. The defense just went all-in with a pair of twos. Merlin has a full-house. They don't know about the bomb that's about to be dropped. They have no idea what the motion is about. The judge hasn't yet shared it with them. The discovery process has been going on for almost a year. Riverside Health kept dragging it out. They thought Merlin would get bored and throw in the towel. They thought they'd wear him down. They thought he'd go broke having no job and no income while these proceedings progressed. They thought wrong. They didn't know about the friendships and acquaintances Merlin developed over the years. They didn't know there were a few people in

Merlin's corner who could buy and sell Riverside Health System.

Chapter 4

Merlin's having a flashback from over ten years ago. Justin Lawton was a very successful person. He was a self-made multi-millionaire. He made a good return on his investments as a developer. He also made a good return on stock investments. Merlin lived in the Carolinas during Reaganomics and did electrical maintenance at Justin's commercial properties throughout the Carolinas.

Merlin developed a casual friendship with Justin. He installed a remote controlled lighting system on Justin's boat dock at Lake Norman. Justin wanted to be able to turn off his dock lights while boating at night. When he pulled into the dock, he'd hit the button on the remote and his dock lights would turn on. When the job was finished, Justin pulled out his checkbook.

"This one's a freebie. No charge," said Merlin.

"Thank-You. In return, I'd like to offer you a freebie. Invest all you can in the speedway when they go public. Sit on it for ten years. You could end up buying the house next door," said Justin.

"Thanks. I'll do that," replied Merlin.

Merlin didn't have a lot of cash to invest, but he did invest just over three grand. The return was almost thirty grand in less than ten years. If he'd have been able to invest thirty grand, he might now be living in a home along Lake Norman.

Merlin has another flashback. This conversation took place over a year ago.

"Justin, I know I can win. There's no doubt in my mind. I've got a full-house up my sleeve. They've got a pair of deuces. We'll get a larger return than we made on the speedway," says Merlin.

"Tell me the high points. Tell me about your full-house," says Justin.

"I'm going to start out by demanding to represent myself. I'll play dumb. I'll make all kinds of mistakes. I have a friend who's a circuit court judge. You might know him. He's from North Carolina. Jerry Olsen. He's going to assist me behind the scenes. I'll make sure my mistakes are the most-common made by anyone attempting to represent themselves. Just before jury selection, I'll drop the bomb, figuratively speaking. When the bomb drops, I promise there will be a dozen huge law firms begging to represent me and take over the case."

"What do you need from me?" Asked Justin.

"Just enough to live on while it drags out. I have enough to get by for about a year. This company is the largest in the county. They're it's largest employer. They have deep pockets and I think their strategy will be to drag it on and wear me out. They know nobody will hire me, since it will be public knowledge I'm suing them for discrimination. You know me. I'm a simple person. I just need enough to allow me to weather the storm."

"Did you apply for unemployment?" Asked Justin.

"No, I didn't. I was advised not to. It wouldn't have been worth it. To win an unemployment suit, I would have had to divulge enough information to prove discrimination or retribution. It would have played into their hand and set the stage for them to offer me much less by way of an out-of-court settlement, which would require a confidentiality clause. The odds of winning unemployment would have been against me because they would lie and be believed. I can't settle out-of-court. I need it all to go public, due to the 'Whistleblower' topics it addresses," replied Merlin.

"What if it doesn't work out? What if you fail? What if you lose?"

"When the bomb drops, I can promise you victory will follow. If it doesn't, I'll come and work it off. You know I'm good for it," Merlin replied.

Chapter 5

The pre-trial meeting continues. The judge handed the bailiff two folders. The bailiff delivered one to the plaintiff and one to the defendant as the judge began to speak.

"Mr. Angelino, the plaintiff is making a motion for you to remove yourself from these proceedings on the grounds you will be called as a witness," said the judge.

Mr. Angelino reads the motion to himself. The last line of the motion says he wasn't held to the same standard as other employees concerning policies relating to discipline. The remaining pages in the folder are copies of his file from Human Resources and a signed agreement relating to the use of a company laptop provided to Mr. Angelino. The file is full of positive entries. The file lists all of his accomplishments as the lawyer for Riverside Health System. There's nothing negative in the file.

"On what grounds? What possible reason would there be for me to be called as a witness? I'm looking at my HR record, but I don't see anything which would exclude me from representing Riverside Health System. I've never had any disciplinary actions taken against me. This doesn't make any sense," says the attorney.

"Mr. Waltz, could you explain what this is about?" Asks the judge.

"Your honor, it's not about what's in the file, it's about what's not in the file. This is about two statements I made in the comments section of the Online Survey. I stated discipline is not properly or fairly administered by IT Management. I also stated IT Management does what they want, if they want, how they want, and for who they want. Mr. Angelino signed a laptop user agreement. In the agreement, it states only he will use the laptop. It also states no software is to be installed on the laptop unless approved and installed by the IT Department. Mr. Angelino violated the agreement and there's no record of a reprimand or even a warning in his HR record," replies Merlin.

"Your honor, I don't recall what the plaintiff is referring to," says the attorney.

"You don't recall work order number 763495? It's the one where you brought your laptop to the IT Department because it wasn't functioning correctly. The tech who did the repair is waiting outside to testify about that work order," replied Merlin.

"Your honor, I object. This has nothing to do with the case at hand," replied Mr. Angelino.

"Mr. Waltz? How does this apply to the case at hand?" Asked the judge.

"It's simple your honor. I think it's what you call fruit from the poisonous tree. People in this company were written up and fired for lesser offenses involving computer usage. When this fact becomes known, they will have the right to sue for wrongful dismissal, mental anguish, pain and suffering, reimbursement for unemployment which was denied because of said discrimination, for one thing. This relates to my statement about IT management doing pretty much whatever they wanted. It's part of the pattern. It helps me to prove my comment in the Online Survey. I intend to show this pattern of doing whatever they wanted extended to advancement being denied, among other things," replied Merlin.

"I see your point. Fruit from the poisonous tree. It's been a while since I heard that one in my courtroom," said the judge.

"Your honor, you're not seriously considering approving this motion?" Asked the attorney.

"Not until I hear all of the evidence. Bailiff, bring in the witness to be sworn," said the judge.

Merlin is now wearing a huge crap-eating grin. He knows he's going to have his motion granted. He's all but busting out with laughter as he recalls the crap-eating grin on his former manager's face while telling him: "If you want to make more money, go get a job down the hill." One good crap-eating grin certainly deserves another. The bailiff leaves the judge's chambers to get Randy Chester. Everybody present can't help but notice the crap-eating grin Merlin has on his face. Even the bailiff noticed it. After the bailiff leaves, the CEO makes a phone call. There's a whispered discussion between the CEO and Mr. Angelino. Mr. Angelino addresses the judge.

"Your honor, with your permission I wish to remove myself from this case. I made a mistake. I was not reprimanded for said mistake. I won't lie. If this goes to trial, I will testify if needed. We'd like to have a fifteen minute recess in order for my client to discuss a possible settlement offer with Mr. Waltz," said Mr. Angelino.

The bailiff returns with Randy Chester. The judge speaks up.

"Mr. Chester, your testimony will not be needed today. This matter has been resolved. You will be required to make yourself available to testify if this matter goes to trial. Is that understood?" Asks the judge.

"Yes, your honor. I live in another area now, but Merlin has my number and knows my current address," replies Randy.

"Let's take a fifteen minute recess," says the judge. Then he continues: "Mr. Angelino, you won't be able to be present during this discussion. Mr. Hocks, I'm going to recommend you secure council before discussing a settlement offer with Mr. Waltz," says the judge.

The CEO reads a text from his phone before responding.

"Your honor, in that case, I'll take your suggestion. Could I possibly request a two hour recess? I have an attorney willing to assist with this matter and his office is just a few blocks away. If Mr. Waltz would be willing to accompany me, we'll go there now to discuss the matter," says the CEO.

"Agreed. We'll meet back here in two hours," said the judge.

Merlin walks alongside the CEO. Once they're outside the courthouse, the CEO speaks up.

"I'd like to hire you back. I'd like this mess to go away. I'd like to make it right. Forgive me for not taking you seriously when this mess started. How about this? I'll pay you for the back pay you were denied and I'll offer you twenty-five percent of the amount you listed for mental anguish and pain and suffering. I'll also terminate your former manager. It sounds to me like he should be the one held most accountable for this situation. I'll give you a total re-instatement and the title and salary you deserve. As I recall, you only had a month or so to go until you hit the four-weeks a year vacation mark. This way, you'll get those four weeks vacation a year. I know you have a chance at winning this case. I won't deny it. But, you should consider juries aren't handing out huge awards like they did fifteen or twenty years ago. You might win and end up with less than what

I'm offering. What are your thoughts about this offer?"

"What about confidentiality? If I accept this offer, am I to assume I'll have to sign a confidentiality agreement?"

"Yes, Merlin. That would be part of the deal," replied the CEO.

"But that would only apply until the company fails, if it fails. I personally think it's destined to fail. What happens then? I'll probably end up out on the street shortly after you get taken over. I'd be surprised if I didn't."

"As CEO, I can assure you I have no intention of seeing this company fail."

"I think it's already heading there. I don't think there's anything you can do to stop it. You see, this company has taken on more debt than it should have. The board of directors were so obsessed with this big new building getting built they couldn't see the forest because of the trees. They were so busy deciding they could, when they should have been asking themselves if they should," replied Merlin.

"You have to understand I had no control over the decision to build and expand."

"You know what really sucks about this mess? I'll tell you. If the head of HR would have been paying attention and doing his job, this whole mess could have been avoided. If the VP would have done her job and did what she said she'd do, this whole mess could have been avoided. If you would have listened to me and did what I requested before I resigned, this whole mess could have been avoided. If you wouldn't have enticed me to stay there with the promise of better advancement opportunities, then welched on the deal, this whole mess wouldn't have happened. Terminating my former manager isn't enough. You can't save your face and your tail at the same time. I told you before I resigned there would be no backing down once I filed suit. This isn't just about me. It's about others. Others who were screwed over and discriminated against and aren't even aware of it. You had your shot. Now, I'm gonna have mine. No deals, no settlement," said Merlin, as he turned and walked away.

Chapter 6

They return to the judges chambers and inform the judge they weren't able to reach an agreement. Riverside Health has a new attorney representing them. They ask for a ninety day continuance so the new attorney can be brought up to speed. Nature of the beast. This is how big business grinds away at the little person. They drag it out as long as they can. People come and go but big business outlives them all. It's the true nature of the beast. This beast is about to be tamed. They're about to get a surprise.

"We will continue in ninety days. Mark your calendars gentlemen," said the judge.

"Your honor, I would like to respectfully request the continuance be extended for six months," replied Merlin.

"Does the defendant have any objections?" Asks the judge.

"No objections, your honor," replied the new attorney for the defendants.

The defense was just played for a fool. They don't even realize what they did. Their view was to drag things out as long as possible. This delay will give Merlin much more time to find a real law firm to represent him. Considering he won a motion to dismiss their own lawyer from the case, he's sure he'll be able to recruit and retain one of the best law firms in the country. That's his goal because he heard somewhere that recruiting and retaining "The Best" is the primary ingredient for a company's success, therefore he thinks it might also be a key ingredient for finding a top-notch law firm in order to win this case.

"Trial to resume with the jury selection starting on February twenty-fourth. We are adjourned," said the judge.

"Wow!" Exclaims Merlin.

"Did you have something to add, Mr. Waltz?" Inquired the judge.

"Sorry for the outburst, your honor. That's my birthday. I'm hoping it's a sign of good luck. I think it's good karma," replied Merlin.

The National Journal is one of the oldest nationwide newspapers in America. Merlin ran a quarter-page ad in the journal for one week. The ad states: "Help. I need a law firm to represent me. I'm in over my head. I have successfully won a motion to have the defense attorney removed from the case because I will be calling him as a witness. I did this while representing myself, but I feel I need a much more knowledgeable and competent law firm to represent me for the remainder of the proceedings. The trial begins in six months. It's an employment discrimination suit with whistleblower ramifications. Other suits will no doubt be brought after this trial is over. There will be no out-of-court settlement. If you are one of the law firms who previously refused to represent me before this trial began, please don't bother offering now. You had your shot." Merlin's contact information is listed at the bottom.

Merlin sent copies of this ad to various local newspapers and television news stations. Not a single one of them responded or acknowledged it. Merlin suspects it's because nobody had the guts to give this hospital bad press. He also suspects it's because this hospital, like many other large hospitals throughout the area, spends millions per year on advertising with them. They'd rather keep the income stream than report the truth. That's ok with Merlin. When this trial is over, he won't offer these local news agencies any interviews or information. He'll only speak to the largest ones. He'll only speak to the "Big Four." This way, no local news agency will be able to hide the truth from the public. Over half of the population watches one of the Big Four news networks, which means over half of the local population will learn the truth.

Chapter 7

A week later, a business meeting is taking place on the eightieth floor of the Sears tower in Chicago. Bentley and Morgan is one of the nation's largest law firms specializing in various types of class-action suits, including employee discrimination. They're one of the firms you see running nationwide ads inviting various people to join their group of plaintiffs.

The conference room is like any other. A few paintings on one wall, a projector screen on another wall, the third wall is covered in dry-erase boards, and the fourth wall is all windows which face the lake. A long table sits in the middle. It seats eighteen people. Jeffery (Jeff) Bentley sits in a seat at one end of the table and Susan Morgan sits in the seat at the other end. They discuss status updates of various cases and various other topics like billing, accounts receivables, expenses, and monthly bonuses. This firm prefers to hold its meetings near the end of the day.

"Is there any new business?" Asks Susan Morgan.

The table is silent. It looks like the meeting will end a little early this week. It only looks that way.

"Did any of you read the National Journal this week?" Asks Jeff Bentley.

"I read it on Sundays," says Jack Wilson, an attorney who just recently joined the firm.

"There's an advertisement in there from a man in Pennsylvania looking for a law firm to represent him in a discrimination suit. He claims he won a motion to have the defendant's lawyer removed because he'll be calling him as a witness. He also claims there will be no out-of-court settlement and other suits will no doubt be brought. His name caught my eye. Merlin Waltz, from Williamsport, Pa. Not often I see or hear the name Merlin. Not often for an individual with no attorney to have such a motion granted. I think it might be worth a follow-up," says Jeff Bentley. Randy Finch, a lawyer whose been with the firm for just over a year, responds.

"I know him. That's my hometown. I actually used to work with him when we were younger," says Randy.

"How well do you know him?"

"We weren't too close, but I know him well enough to approach him and hold conversation with him," replies Randy.

"Talk about a coincidence. What are the odds? I'm a big believer in karma. Randy, I'd like you to initiate contact. Find out the whole story. Take a look at all of the evidence. Put him at ease.

Something tells me we need to take this case. Get back to me with the details."

"I'm a little concerned about not being able to settle out-of-court. It could translate into a major loss for us," says Susan.

"Yes, there's always that possibility. I suspect there's a good reason. I've never seen a person run an ad in the National Journal to find a law firm. He sounds like he might know a little more about marketing than the average person. Let's get all the details and go from there. We've been lacking a little on pro-bono lately, so maybe this will make up for it. If other cases do develop because of it, it could mean much more in the long run. I'll bet our marketing firm could twist this into something really positive, regardless of the outcome," says Jeff.

A week later, Bentley and Morgan are listed as the firm who will represent Merlin Waltz in his case against Riverside Health System. Bentley and Morgan is one of the top ten firms in the country. They have a ninety-five percent track record for winning. When they heard all of the details about the case, they knew they couldn't turn it down, regardless of the outcome.

Once it became known Bentley and Morgan was on the case, Riverside Health System dumped their local downtown law firm and invested in a large national firm to represent them. Riverside Health

System tried to get a longer delay but the judge denied it. They threatened the possibility of grounds for a mistrial. The judge reminded them they were willing to use the downtown attorney for a possible out-of-court settlement and the discussion between the CEO and Merlin Waltz concerning that settlement would be admissible. The CEO made a mistake trying to make an offer when he didn't have his lawyer present for the discussion. The judge made it clear there would be no mistrial, nor would this be a topic for appeal because they themselves had already asked for and agreed to ninety days to bring their new lawyer up to speed. It was Merlin who asked to extend to six months. Only eight weeks have passed since that time, therefore the defendants still have over ninety days to get their new lawyers up to speed.

In the days to come, many will wonder if Merlin outsmarted them, or did they outsmart themselves? The bottom line is there will be no more delays. The trial will proceed. The date has been set. Merlin is now wearing a very large crap-eating grin.

Chapter 8

The big day is here. It's February twenty-fourth. The trial begins. Randy Finch is representing the plaintiff. It drags on for almost six months. The case has been handed to the jury. The jury was given specific instructions. After nearly two days of deliberations, the bailiff escorted the foreperson, James Dunkelberg, to see the judge. The judge called both attorneys to the bench.

"Mr. Dunkelberg, could you repeat your question? I need both attorneys to hear the question before I issue a response," said the judge.

"Yes, your honor. We want to know if we are allowed to award a higher amount in damages," said the foreperson.

"As jurors, you are permitted to allow as little, or as much in damages as you see fit. You are permitted to allow anything from zero up to whatever amount you feel is proper," replied the judge.

The bailiff escorted Mr. Dunkelberg back to the jury room. Meanwhile, there's a flurry of whispered discussions going on at the defense table. The defense attorney asked for a meeting in chambers to discuss a settlement offer.

"If said offer involves signing a non-disclosure agreement or a confidentiality agreement, there will be no offer accepted," said Randy Finch.

There's nothing worse than being between a rock and a hard place. The defense wants to settle, but they don't want to admit any wrong-doing. The jury awards Merlin double the amount he was asking for. The news is on all of the worldwide networks. In an interview with BNN, Merlin made it clear if the CEO would have done what should have been done, Merlin would still be working there and multiple managers would have been put out on the street. When this story aired, the CEO retired. He claimed the recent years of local expansion and change was too much of a demand on him. When asked if the board requested he resign, he said: "No, not at all." Many speculate he was asked to step down, but when the board was asked about it, they said: "No comment."

Merlin was interviewed on "Talk Tonight," one of the nightly talk shows with the BNN News Network. When asked why he wouldn't settle out of court, he replied: "Multiple reasons. Number one: This mess could have been avoided. Number two: Had I settled, a confidentiality clause would have prohibited multiple others from learning the truth. That truth being, they could bring a viable and winnable discrimination suit against this hospital, based on evidence admitted during my case. Number three: I'm going to write a book and a screenplay about this experience and, since it's based on the truth, I'm sure I'll make a decent profit between the book and movie rights."

A class action suit was brought against Riverside Health by Bentley and Morgan. It went on for over two years. The total awards were over sixty million. Riverside Health went into receivership. Shortly afterwards, a former competitor less than sixty miles away, took control of Riverside Health. They eliminated the local Board of Directors. They also eliminated twenty-five percent of the managers. They increased the starting pay for unskilled employees to eleven dollars an hour.

Merlin had great success with his book sales while the class-action suit was going on. Riverside Health tried to get a gag order against Merlin, but they failed. His book was true, and they had no grounds for a gag order. While Riverside was busy fighting the class-action, Merlin worked on the screenplay. After it was announced Riverside Health was going into receivership, Merlin sold the screenplay and the movie rights for an undisclosed amount. Guess who's now wearing the biggest crap-eating grin you ever saw in your life?

Chapter 9

I wish I could tell you Chapters three through eight were true. I'm very sorry to say they are not true. I will tell you they could have been true, but sometimes life has a way of throwing you an unexpected curve now and then. I wanted to add a little excitement and drama to the story with the hope you might be encouraged to read the rest of the story. If not, I totally understand. Some will find the real story to be a bit boring at times and may think it's in poor taste. It does have some humor and drama but, most of all, it has the truth. It also has the potential of opening the flood gates for hundreds of millions in losses, litigation, or exposure. So, If you think you can handle the truth, please continue reading. The real story starts here.

My first position in the IT field was with a company doing residential cable-modem installations in the mid nineties. I worked in an area which was a Beta territory. It was a very good transitional position. They needed people who could do physical cabling for the home-networking needs and do the software and hardware installations on the computer. I gained exposure and experience in cutting-edge technology during that time.

Later on, I accepted a position in the IT Department at a Hospital in Pennsylvania. There were two divisions in the department, and over 50 employees in the department at the time. By Health Care standards, this company was also considered cutting-edge. They were a Beta site for a very large software vendor. A variety of systems were brought live at this facility with the purpose of attracting new customers to the vendor.

In preparing for an upcoming change to a web-based Financial and Clinical system, it was discovered they needed to find a way to automate the deployment process of various types of software relating to the live event. There were constant changes and many various needs relating to software deployment. Otherwise, they would have to send all of the techs out to do the installations via "Sneaker Net." Sneaker Net wasn't anything covert or sneaky. It's the term used when you have to physically walk to a computer, sit down in front of it, sign in with the proper credentials, and then do the installation. If you have over 1,500 computers to visit, this would be a lot of work, especially if you needed to do it multiple times during the preparation of a massive system implementation. Even with remote connection software, it would take a very long time. I ended up being the person who learned how to setup and configure various types of software to be automatically deployed with no user-intervention required.

I was the only person in the entire department who held a Professional Certification from Microsoft. I had one previously to accepting employment there, but it had expired. I updated my certification by obtaining the most recent one, at the time, for Windows XP. The certification exams are broken up into five different areas of expertise. On the security portion, I achieved a 100%. I then went on to achieve status as a Systems Administrator - MCSA. To achieve this, I was required to pass three more exams. On all three of those exams, I achieved 100% in the security section. I then went on to achieve status as a Systems Engineer - MCSE. Really cool, eh? No, I'm not Canadian; but I like a little Canadian humor now and then. And, I wanted to make sure you were still awake. Obtaining my Systems Engineering certification required passing three more exams. I scored 100% on all of the remaining security sections. I passed a total of seven exams and received a 100% grade on the security portion for every single one of them. Was this a coincidence? Who knows. Maybe I just had a natural gift from above when it came to understanding security and the nature of it. I always made sure my manager was aware of this fact. One typically didn't achieve 100% in more than one area, and these exams were very complicated. To achieve a 100% in the same section on all seven exams would be rare indeed. Not unheard of, but rare. It should have been a sign to my manager Security might be a good fit for me moving forward. But, sometimes managers really don't care about your future. Sometimes, they're more concerned about playing politics. Sometimes, managers are sadists who abuse their position and the control they have over the destinies of others.

Whenever I decided to learn something, I always did it hands-on. Maybe it's because I attended a

Trade School during high school and it's how I was formally taught. I liked it better that way. I found it easier to learn something when I could read about it and do it at the same time. That's what worked for me. So, while studying for my various certifications, I learned it hands-on. I set up multiple servers. I installed and configured all of the various servers as I read and learned about them. I installed an Active Directory, an SQL Database server, an Email server, a Backup system, a Web server with multiple web-sites and web-based applications, just to name a few. Basically, my data-center was the same as what was used in the company where I worked, it was just smaller. I also used this home network in order to learn more about software deployment and security. Software deployment has very few formal certifications available. There are companies who will certify you on their particular system or their unique software, but in the real world, you usually need to know a lot about various kinds of software to do software deployment.

I was "The Man" when it came to software deployment. I created the customized executable files, the customized registry settings, and designed the proper process for each deployment. There were times when I would thoroughly test something, and once the live deployment started, an unknown or unexpected problem appeared. There's always a percentage of failure. The goal is to have a low percentage of failure and minimize impact to the end-users when failures occur. If there are major

Merlin Waltz

problems affecting the end-users, the Service Center would be swamped with calls.

I spent close to ten years at this company. I prefer to call it a decade. If you consider the hours I worked, and the amount of personal time I invested, it was definitely over a decade. I saw many changes. I experienced some good things and some bad things. Here are some interesting facts pertaining to this department and my work history during the time I was there. I was never written-up. I never received a verbal or written warning. My attendance was average. I worked more overtime than anyone in the entire department. I might have even worked more overtime than anyone in the entire company during my time there. I don't know for sure, but I'm sure I was in the top five, when considering hourly employees who weren't in a direct patient-support role, such as the nursing department.

The company had over 2,000 employees at the time. Once in a while, there would be newly created positions with titles which previously hadn't existed. One example would be a Physician's Assistant (PA), another would be a Hospitalist. Naturally, there was employee turnover. Various people left from various departments and from a variety of disciplines ranging from Management to Unit Clerks. There were also some who left the IT Department, accepting opportunities elsewhere. A Vice-President, A physician with the title of CMIO (Corporate Medical Information Officer), three or four managers and seven or eight hourly employees left the department during my time there. They all gave a two-week notice, did their two weeks, and moved on. When I decided to move on, I also gave a two-week notice.

I was very involved with the largest and most important software deployment ever completed to date. It was a major version upgrade to the clinical and pharmacy system. These types of upgrades are usually nick-named "forklift" upgrades, because you almost need a forklift to remove the old servers and install the new ones. Some updates or upgrades are just minor changes and sometimes the equivalent of putting "Lipstick on a pig." That's where the back-end of the system looks and operates the same, but the user interface is a little fancier. I'm having a little laugh as I recall an old saying: "You can put a pig in a tuxedo and take it out to dinner at a fancy restaurant, but it will still be a pig."

A manager with the company's primary software vendor (and one of the largest in the health care industry) was so impressed with what I did, he expressed interest in the possibility of having me do a presentation at a worldwide event that year in Las Vegas. The event in Las Vegas was where the Vendor showcased the best of the best to the entire world. People from a variety of healthcare disciplines attended. People came from all over the world. Most of them were doctors and managers. Before the end of my two weeks, I was asked to stay another week by my manager. I'm sure some of you are wondering why. The answer is obvious. Nobody in the IT Department or the entire company could do the job I was doing. But, if nobody else could do the job, wouldn't the average person think it should be a fairly secure position by way of title and compensation? Yes, the average person of average intelligence would think so, but that was not the case. I like the sound of that. I feel it needs to be repeated: The average person of average intelligence would think so, but that was not the case. How about we put that another way: A tenth grader might think so, but there's never a tenth grader around when you need one.

How many people have you met in your life who were asked to stay an extra week, after giving a two-week notice in any position at any company? Have you ever met one? The ones I found via internet searching shared they stayed reluctantly, because of concerns about a future reference from their employer. Of course, I stayed the extra week. How nice to have it on my resume. How nice to know four or five managers, six or eight hourly employees, a doctor with the title of CMIO, and a Vice President all departed the IT Department at the end of their two-week notice, and I was being asked to stay another week. I wonder how many other employees in the entire company were asked to stay an extra week after giving their two-week notice during the time I was employed there, and what their salary and title was? It would be interesting to know the answer to that question. I wonder if it's in my employee file at the HR department. I wonder if HR ever knows an employee has given a two-week notice. I wonder. I wander. I wonder. I wander.

I wonder if you knew, Mr. CEO, I worked a lot of overtime during my years there. I also worked a lot of overtime during my last two years there. Wasn't there supposed to be no overtime when the new building project started? I recall something about saving money and being good financial stewards and one of the ways of doing it was to eliminate all overtime, unless it related directly to patient care? I guess my manager didn't hear what I heard. Or, maybe it was just a rumor and I totally misunderstood it's meaning. You see, I don't have a four-year degree, so maybe I have a diminished ability to understand things at that level.

I was sitting in the cafeteria on the last Friday of my employment there. Not my last day, but my last Friday. You see, I was going to be working the weekend to complete the major system migration at Saturday midnight. By the way, Mr. CEO, how many people worked overtime during their last two weeks of employment there? I'd like to know. Anyhow, back to the incident at hand. I was eating lunch when the director of the software division stopped by. He gave me some cock and bull story about how it was a shame I was leaving, while all the while wearing a nice big crap-eating grin. I asked him if he was aware the manager with our vendor was so impressed with my software deployment work he wanted me to host a seminar in

Las Vegas that year. He responded by saying: "Well, you have to work in Healthcare to do that," and then he turned and walked away very quickly. They like to stick the knife in your back, then twist it. Under normal circumstances, I would have expected a person in his position to say something like: "Gee, Merlin - I'm surprised your manager didn't try to retain you." or "This is very important and glorifying news, Merlin. Has your manager attempted to retain you? The CEO and the Marketing department would be very impressed about this." It's a shame that neither of the previous statements were made. He did what this department's managers were famous for. Don't ask, don't tell. Pretend it isn't happening. Don't acknowledge the fact someone who works under you might be better and/or smarter than you. You see, Mr. CEO, this is one of the main reasons some of the best people who worked in your IT Department are no longer there.

I wonder if there's any information on record with the Human Resources department about my experience with software deployment. I doubt it. The fact I was one of a small percentage in the entire IT field nationwide with over five years of knowledge and experience as a software deployment specialist (at that time) was not on record at HR, nor was it known to HR. If it was, then somebody at HR was sleeping at the wheel. It should have been, but it wasn't. A lot went on in this department that wasn't on the record or known to the Human Resources department. There was a lot that went on in this department the CEO didn't know about. This story will explain a little bit about why. It will also be providing some information which was unknown to the Board of Directors, the CEO, HR, Marketing, and to a few others.

The local newspaper has a professional section where various achievements and accomplishments are displayed for all to see. Was my name and picture ever in this professional section? No, it was not. I wonder why? An MCSE certification was one of the most prestigious in the IT field at that time. The average salary was very high. I did some research about various employees who were listed in this section by this company over the years. Do you know what I found? The typical salary of those certifications and/or achievements was much lower than the typical salary of a person with their MCSE. So, why were their pictures, names, and accomplishments posted in the newspaper? Who makes the decision to post them there? I believe it may be the marketing department. I wonder how it works. I know how it doesn't work. I suspect someone may have inquired about my accomplishments and they were purposely downplayed by my manager or a member of IT Management in order to keep belittling me and denying me the recognition I deserved. Some say blowing your own horn is egotistical. Others say if you don't blow your own horn, nobody else will. In this department, management was very good at blowing their own horns. I never once saw them blow anyone else's horn, unless it was related to an accomplishment made by another IT manager.

This company had an internal little newspaper which was printed every month. It was distributed throughout the company. Lots of copies. You'd see dozens of them on the tables in the cafeteria and almost every sitting area or waiting room in the company. When I achieved status as an MCSA, there was a write-up placed there by my manager. It was a decent statement about my accomplishment, but it was no where near what it should have been. I didn't know it at the time, but it was the beginnings of multiple retaliations and retributions which were going to be taken against me. Later, when I achieved status as an MCSE, the story in the company publication was so lame, it was almost as though my manager was telling you I ate oatmeal for breakfast.

Hello, Mr. CEO. What was it you used to say? Some line of bull-squat about the success of the company being based on recruiting and retaining the best people and treating them well? I want to make sure you know there was no attempt to retain me. I want you to know I was not treated well. This is just one example of how various members of IT Management made a bold-faced liar out of you. Multiple managers knew about this situation. Don't ask, don't tell. That was their motto. Pretend it isn't really happening. Play dumb. If I was a manager and knew of an employee who had accomplished so much, I would have immediately reported it to the

CEO. This story will show you some of the reasons why I was never considered for management and why a proper position and salary was never created for me.

The IT Department used to sub-contract their services to other hospitals. This allowed these other hospitals to operate with lower overhead relating to their IT support. The manager from the software vendor told me and the IT Clinical Manager that he had hospitals screaming at him for help and assistance to deploy this software. This was during a conference call relating to the upgrade we were working on. Not a single IT Manager cared about this statement. They could have worked out arrangements to have me work as a consultant at other hospitals to help them to get the current upgrade deployed. I could have made your company millions of dollars in revenue, and a major percentage of the revenue would have been profit. But they would have had to pay me what I was worth. They couldn't do that. That would mean they would have to eat crow. They'd rather screw the company out of millions in revenue than pay me what I was worth. If any of those managers read this and say something like: "Gee, we never thought of that," I would suggest they be fired on the spot. Such an idiotic statement is not acceptable to me. If they never thought of that, then they are all total idiots and shouldn't be employed there. They couldn't be that stupid, especially since one of them was on the front-cover of a trade publication with a story about their success at offering IT support to other hospitals. Another one of them was quoted within the article relating to the cover story. I'm wondering if HR or the CEO knew I already saved the IT department over half a million dollars in direct labor during the years I did software deployment. That's right. If multiple techs would have had to do what I did all by myself for over five years, over half a million would have been spent on labor alone, and that's not counting the overhead of management's involvement or the numerous calls which would have been made to the service center. And a majority of this work would have to be done on overtime. Some of it would have been done during normal hours, but considering we were understaffed by a minimum of three field techs, (In my opinion) a majority of it would have been done on overtime.

A few people were surprised when they saw me there for a third week. Some asked why, and some of them knew why. After my initial resignation was made known to the entire department, seven out of ten employees informed me I was lucky to be getting out of there, or words to that effect. Seventy percent, and just in case anybody is wondering, it was seventy percent of the entire department. And when I say the entire department, I'm talking about both divisions. I'm talking about the entire department. I don't mean to imply there was a management problem within the department; I mean to state there most definitely was a management problem. But there was one awesome person in management. If I had worked for that manager, I might still be there today. Who knows? But, concerning certain managers who have control over people's titles, salaries, retirements, vacations, pensions, career paths, and futures, I would say there clearly was a problem. The biggest problem was nobody was watching the watchdogs. The foxes were watching the chickens in the pen; The problem was nobody watched them. And these were some pretty sly foxes, or so they thought. I'm betting they never expected to see their magnificent accomplishments made public. Let's see how sly they were. A secret is only kept if it's never made public.

I've got a secret. I'm no longer going to keep it a secret. I'm going to share it with the world. Most of the world won't care. Most of the world will never read this story. But it will be available for all eternity. Almost every word ever written or spoken publicly since the dawn of the twentieth century is on record for all of humanity to read.

Chapter 10

I started out with the title of PC Technician. I was always very gifted at trouble-shooting and problem solving. Within my first sixty days I became the Project Team Leader. However, there was no real title or position for that job, nor was there a proper pay level. It didn't concern me. I'm one who prefers to ask for what I deserve when I have no doubt in my mind I deserve it. A little later I was given a different title and a raise in pay for over-seeing the project team. The project team was responsible for installing various upgrades to systems and new system implementations; they were also responsible for new PC installations and replacements when needed.

When I first went to work for the company, they were getting ready to expand the IT Department. This was due to a support contract being entered into with another company. That company would eliminate their IT Department and this company would take care of their IT support. Two people from that company became employees of this one. One was made a manager over the Service Center and another was on the service team I was overseeing. The conversion to all of the new systems involved multiple hardware and software changes. After this internal department expansion, my manager was promoted to a director's position. I guessed with the added duties and responsibilities and additional employees under him, somebody felt it was appropriate. That's how it works at the top.

At the bottom it works a little differently, as you'll soon learn. But there was one glimmer of hope: My manager always said there was money in the budget for advancement, all you needed to do was get certified. He said this repeatedly for over two years. I had two certifications under my belt, and made it clear to my manager I was going to get two more and achieve status as an MCSA. I also explained I was going to continue forward and get my MCSE.

Then, a funny thing happened. A few weeks later, we were in a network division meeting. Someone mentioned they thought we should be paid more. My manager responded by saying: "There's always money in the budget for advancement. We'll put you on a two-year plan." How interesting. All of the sudden, when an employee is halfway to attaining his MCSA, and planning to have it in about six months, it's announced there's something called a two-year plan? How convenient. This so-called two year plan had never been mentioned prior to that day. Nor had it ever been mentioned during any of my yearly performance reviews. Don't you think that's funny? Come on now. I told you this was a humorous story. You're supposed to be laughing.

A funny thing happened during the first large project I was overseeing. I was the person doing most of the work. It was a very hectic schedule. I was also the person who worked the most overtime. Moving forward, this became the standard for me. It was a constant juggling of schedules, deadlines, disasters, and politics. In over nine years with this company, I can only recall one time when somebody was told: "No, we're sorry but you will have to wait." There were also times when we would do an installation exactly according to the specifications and information provided, only to find out a major change was needed because we weren't provided with the proper information. Did this change the deadline or the live date? No, it did not. Did anyone else ever have their feet held to the fire for making such mistakes? I'm sure you already know the answer. Just wing an email, cc a few managers and a VP or two, and things just magically happen.

And what happened to the projects which were already scheduled? We would just contact certain people and explain we needed to push back the schedule. Of course, I was the person who did this on many occasions. The people who were patient, organized, and understanding would be put on the back burner for those who were not patient, organized, or understanding. I was one who always pushed for more understanding of what it really takes to properly complete an installation from start to finish. Unfortunately, my experience and opinions were never taken seriously. In my opinion, unless a major amount of savings or revenue was going to be created by changing project priorities, somebody should have been saying "No." Do you know how much time is wasted by way of inefficiency when you start multiple projects, then put them on a back burner to return to later?

Answer: A lot. Do you want it done properly, or do you want it done fast? Politics were more important than efficiency.

Chapter 11

A person had left the service center and the open position was posted. The manager of the service center (we'll call him Joe) was interviewing new applicants. One day, a department email came from Joe announcing a candidate had accepted the open position. A short time after that, a position was posted for a person who would be involved with obtaining various grants for the company. The service center manager (we'll call him Joe) accepted this position. A short time later, I was in a meeting with my manager and I was informed he had Joe removed as the service center manager because he made the decision to hire the new service center rep without permission. I thought this was very strange. Joe was a manager. It seemed strange to me his job description wouldn't have included that responsibility. I looked up the job description. I won't tell you what it said. I don't think I need to.

I always wondered why I was told about this fact? I wasn't a manager. I wasn't a supervisor. I wasn't a member of the club. It just didn't sit well with me. It was almost as if my manager was informing me: "I am in control, and I can do whatever I want to do." I didn't bother to ask my manager why he was telling me this. I already knew why. It was because he didn't want me to apply for the position. What other possible reason could there be? He had already decided who was getting the position. The problem is you made one mistake, Mr.

Manager. You told me. Don't worry, I got the hint. I wasn't planning to apply for the job. I had no interest in applying for the job. I felt there were others more deserving of the opportunity. And, after what I just learned, I knew I wouldn't have the autonomy or the support of IT Management to make the service center what it truly could and should be. You'd rather play politics than do right by your employees. That's my personal opinion. Concerning Joe's replacement, I know one person who applied for the job had management experience and had been there longer than I. This person didn't get the job and I truly feel it was because of a disagreement or misunderstanding which happened with someone in IT Management in the recent past. I won't go into details. I'll save it for the movie. I also know of another person who had been there longer and had expressed interest in the position. I don't know if he actually applied for the position or not, but he didn't get it.

I achieved my goal of obtaining my Systems Administrator certification. During that time, and prior to getting this certification, something happened in the IT Department. A bunch of employees gave negative feedback on the Online Survey. This didn't surprise me. And what happened in the following year didn't surprise me. I won't waste time here going into detail about the questions on the survey. That will be much better portrayed in the movie. In a staff meeting, the VP stated: "IT Management is taking these survey results very serious, and we're going to address all of these issues." The keyword is: All. But it didn't happen. What happens to Vice-Presidents who lie through their teeth? They retire with honors, of course. What happens to the employees who then had retribution taken against them because they were honest on the Online Survey? A majority of them left the company. One of them left the company and wrote a book about it. Can you guess who it is? Can you guess who's laughing now?

Management did what they had been doing all along. They did whatever they wanted. The VP hid out in her glass-castle of an office and buried her head in the sand like an ostrich. Big Bird. That was the nickname I gave her. I never told anyone in the network division about the nickname I gave her. To my knowledge, the network division (collectively) had no nickname for her. Until now, nobody ever knew I gave her the nickname of Big Bird. I kept it a secret. Until now. In the software support division her nickname was "Witch-Bitch." I always wondered why they gave her such a nickname. I never cared enough to find out, but I heard her referred to as the "Witch-Bitch" by a majority of the employees in the software division. It's kind of ironic when you think about it. This division was looked upon by IT Management as "better than." "Better than" the network division. No employee in the software division ever acted "better than." No employee from the software division ever treated any employee from the network division as though they were "less than." It was IT Management, collectively, who considered them better, and considered our division less than, or less important. I hope you find this funny. I certainly did. Are you laughing? You should be. Come on! Where's your sense of humor? Isn't it comical to learn the division who was considered "better than" by management nicknamed the VP "The Witch-Bitch?" and the "less than" division didn't even have a nickname for her? I think it's quite ironic and hilarious. I know I'm laughing.

So, the Vice-President fluffed the problem off on the problem. In other words, she let the managers who worked for her address the issues. In hindsight, what she really did, was involve herself in a conspiracy. When she fluffed the problem off on the problem, she became a part of the problem. So, her subordinates put on a dog-and-pony show. They held meetings and gave everyone a few free lunches and listened to input and feedback relating to the various questions which were asked on the survey. They never asked about the comments section of the survey. The comments were never brought up for discussion. Various employees were very unhappy about this, including myself. If a survey has an open-ended comment box for input, the input should have been talked about. It was part of the survey. Not that it mattered, because management had absolutely no intentions of doing anything about anything, unless they wanted to. One manager even stated: "Nothing is going to change because IT Management doesn't want anything to change." My manager had been talking about re-organizing his division for years. For over eight years, it was just talk. Nothing ever happened. The only words out of this manager's mouth during this Online Survey fiasco was that he needed to get the re-org completed. He said it many times. He said it many ways. It was his way of holding power and control over the employees. During that year, the word "re-org" was mentioned more times than one could ever imagine. Numerous employees were wondering why management never addressed any issues. Time was dragging on, and the next survey wasn't too far away. Not a single new policy was created. Not a single methodology was changed. A couple very minor issues were addressed, but they were very minor. They were very low in priority. They were only done so management could delude themselves into thinking they did what they said would be done.

The sad part is a majority of the questions on the survey relate to management. I wonder how many other companies are run in this way? I wonder if all companies let the problem take care of the problem? Does anyone realize if the survey process is corrupted, your company is corrupted and your company is not a so-called "best employer" or "best place" to work for?

Management did something else during this time. They treated everyone in the department with more kindness than was ever thought possible. They would bend over to be kind to the employees. They handed out more free lunch passes than ever before. A manager had the ability to give an employee a free lunch pass as a way of showing appreciation for going the extra mile in certain situations. They were so nice during that one year, it sometimes made you want to puke your guts out in the nearest toilet, or in some cases, you might want to puke so fast you had to keep it from hitting your own shoes because you couldn't get to a bathroom quick enough. That's how some people react to a dog-and-pony show. Especially when they know it's a dog-and-pony show, and everyone knew it was a dog-and-pony show. I was so sickened by seeing all of this faked kindness that I myself considered shoving my fingers down my throat to induce vomiting more times than I can remember.

Everyone's questions were answered at the announcement of the next survey. Management had gotten the survey broken down into multiple sections for the next Online Survey. This was by design. This was part of the conspiracy which took place. The previous survey was not done by sections, or divisions. It was one survey, with one web-link the entire department used. This time would be different. This time, it would be done by sections and divisions.

It was the head manager of the software division who emailed the entire department informing everyone to be sure they were using the correct survey link. He sent the email multiple times. I believe he sent it more than five times. A majority of the employees were intimidated by this. What could they do? They couldn't go to the VP. Big

Bird wouldn't have listened. She couldn't have heard anything if she was listening because her head was buried in the sand. To give negative feedback would do them no good. They already knew it would do no good. The proof was right in front of them. It was almost as though management was saying: "We dare you to give negative feedback. If you do, we'll know where it came from, which section, and who to come down on." Everyone got the hint. Everyone understood. What could they do? It was apparent management was going to continue doing things their way, and they did. My question: Why didn't the VP send this email? Shouldn't an email which affected the entire department, meaning all divisions and sections, have been sent by the VP? I'll tell you why. She was busy making sure her head stayed in the sand, and she couldn't reach the keyboard to type the email.

It's my opinion this company did not deserve the award for "Best State Employer" from this point forward. It's my opinion all of the survey results were tainted, moving forward, due to what happened while I worked there. If a company wants to brag about being a "Best Employer" to work for, they should not leave it up to management to address issues relating to negative feedback on these surveys. Most of the questions on the survey related to management. If there's a problem with management, who should address it? I think HR should address it. It's my opinion allowing the problem to fix the problem is not the answer. The discrimination, unfair treatment, denial of proper advancement, and retribution taken against me, and others, are just a few reasons why.

When I had my next performance review, I said I'd like to know how my MCSA certification would affect my future. I thought it would mean something to be the first person there to have an MCSA. I thought wrong. My manager informed me there was no money in the budget for advancement, and if I wanted a raise, I should go get a job down the hill. While he was telling me this, he was wearing a nice big crap-eating grin. The term "down the hill" referred to the other division in the IT Department. It was the same as saying: "You're never getting squat from me." He didn't see the big picture. He didn't realize the conspiracy he was involved in could open up the company to multiple millions in losses, litigation, and exposure, if anyone went public. He portrayed the attitude which was felt and shared by many employees in this company: "We're the biggest employer in the area and we know it. If you're not happy, you should leave."

I got the message loud and clear. My manager was taking retaliation and retribution against me because I was honest on the Online Survey. No problem. I can handle it. I'd rather be honest. I have more integrity. I knew the day would come when the truth would be known. I didn't know at the time it would be me exposing it. I kept my chin up and continued with my certification studies.

Chapter 12

I went to see the manager of the Service Center one afternoon. The manager was doing some paperwork when I entered his office. He informed me he was doing something he'd never done before: He was writing someone up. He then went on to tell me he was being very careful about it because the man was black, and was married to a white woman, and he needed to ensure he did it properly. Can you believe this? Why would he tell me such a thing? Why would he say such a thing? The answer is simple: As a member of management, he was showing me he could do anything he wanted, say anything he wanted, and if it got ugly, he would be believed because he was a member of management. I was suppressing a grin while I imagined a turkey strutting his stuff. I was also grinning to myself while remembering the hiring of this black man was the reason the previous Service Center manager was removed from the position. I also realized this company had very few black people in it, by comparison, and I couldn't recall a single black person in upper-management. Maybe there was, but I surely don't recall one. I can tell you there definitely was never a black person in IT Management while I was there.

Is this a coincidence? You tell me. I worked in this department for almost ten years. During that time, one black person was hired. Only one. And this was in a department of about fifty employees. And the man who hired him got removed from his position for hiring him. I heard a rumor that years earlier there was another black man who worked there, but I don't know how long he worked there, nor do I know why he left. But I find it very strange in ten years time, only one black person was hired in this department. In fact, I can only recall one single time a black man was interviewed for a position in this department. Whenever a person was interviewed, they were usually taken around the department and introduced to most of the employees. I was introduced to multiple interviewees, but can only recall one who was black. Part of me wonders if this person was interviewed to keep up appearances. Part of me wonders if the black man who was hired was only interviewed to keep up appearances. Years later, there was one other black person interviewed, but he didn't get the job.

I mentioned to the Service Center manager that I was unhappy about the outcome of my recent performance review. I also mentioned I was tired of the lies, lip-service, and bull-squat I was getting from my manager. I mentioned I was told there was no money in the budget for advancement. I didn't mention the part about being told to go get a job down the hill. I kept that bit of information to myself. I had this manager in a corner. He didn't know what to say. He didn't know what to do. You see, this manager typically had to go to his manager, who was also my manager, on a regular basis in order to function in his position. Many thought this strange. Many thought this was ridiculous. But, as it turns out, I was about to learn the service center manager was a genius. A true genius. A real genius. A super genius. He suggested I should compile a list of reasons, or justifications for obtaining a raise and a promotion. Then, present it to my manager. Then he made a statement about possible outcomes. He said: "Maybe your manager only gives raises to the squeaky wheels. Maybe you should show him why you deserve a raise, and if he disagrees, well then, it is what it is. And, if you decide to leave the company, I'll certainly support you and give you a good reference." Genius. True Genius. This man should be CEO. I would have never thought of such a thing. Here was another example of management flexing their muscles. What I was really being told was: If you don't like it here, then leave. Please note: I don't recall any questions on the Online Survey relating to being a squeaky wheel.

The service center manager was in a jamb when I met with him. He didn't know what to do. He might have been trained about what to do, but the training didn't align with the controlling person he answered to. That's an opinion based on years of experience. You see, he couldn't call daddy for help, because I was complaining about daddy. I'm betting he was probably trained to direct an unhappy employee to HR. He couldn't do that. It would violate the rules. IT Management had their own internal HR department. They were in control. Are you laughing? Remember, this is supposed to be funny. I'm laughing because this manager thought he got away with this stunt. Surprise! You didn't get away with squat. The CEO now knows.

Over the next few months, Mr. Service Center manager had asked me if I had taken his advice. I replied I wasn't going to shake the money tree. I didn't tell him I had come up with a better idea. A funny thing happened a short time later. Another tech passed a certification exam. One exam. Only one. And the tech received a raise and a promotion. The tech was promoted to the same title and rate of pay I was receiving at the time. The hourly pay increase was close to twenty percent. This happened shortly after I was informed there was no money in the budget for advancement. This tech was on the two-year plan which was mentioned earlier. I was the service team leader, with seven techs under me. This tech was also under me. Now, here is the problem. This two-year plan was a scam. Remember: My manager didn't offer to put me on this so-called two-year plan, even after I attained status as an MCSA. He told me to go get a job down the hill if I wanted to make more money. Isn't this discrimination? It is in my book. But my book is based on reality and common sense. My book is based on what is fair, what is right, and what is wrong. A person passes one certification exam and receives nearly twenty percent in pay increase. A person passes four certification exams and receives nothing. Isn't that funny? I'm listening, but I don't hear you laughing yet.

I did a little research. I hung a piece of paper on my office wall. It was a daily reminder which helped me to keep moving forward. It was a listing of salary ranges for people in the area who had their Systems Administrator Certification. Of course, my pay was nowhere near any of them. I hoped the day would come when it would be. Maybe a miracle will happen and somebody will get their head out of the dark. I doubted it, but I didn't give up hope.

Prior to my next performance review, I completed three more certification exams and achieved status as a Certified Systems Engineer - MCSE. I also took the Service Center manager's advice. I did some research and came up with reasons to justify a raise. I also became the squeaky wheel. At my next performance review, I shared some research with my manager concerning software deployment, and titles and salaries related to it. Why did I do that? I did it for a very good reason. The salary range was almost forty percent higher than what the typical Systems Engineer earned. I did not have the title or salary of a Systems Engineer at the time, nor did I have the title or salary of a Software Deployment Specialist, but I was doing the work of one. It was one of the most important hats I wore while I worked there. I had acquired over five years of experience doing it by then. Although I wasn't doing it full-time, I was the only person doing it. I was basically told "thank-you" for providing this information about Software Deployment Specialists, and then I was told achieving status as a Systems Engineer was "Big."

Kind of sounds a little strange, don't you think? I'll bet you're wondering where this is going. This information was not provided to HR as part of my performance review. It should have been, but it wasn't. If it was, then somebody was sleeping at the wheel. My manager placed a statement in my performance review that in the upcoming reorganization, or "re-org" as it had come to be known, there would be a position suitable for me which was going to utilize my knowledge, ability, and experience. Yes, it was going to do just that. As long as I was willing to do it for a lot less pay than I deserved. Was I given a raise for obtaining my MCSE certification? No, I was not. I passed seven certification exams and didn't receive one red cent in salary increase for any of them. Discrimination on parade. I updated the papers hanging on my office wall. I posted a newer one which related to salaries of Systems Engineers in the area. I added a sheet showing salaries relating to Software Deployment Specialists.

Chapter 13

Every year during the Christmas season, the CEO visited various departments. Something odd happened on his next Christmas visit. I got sent off on a wild goose chase just prior to his arrival. I didn't know it at the time. I didn't know he was on his way. I was sent out to take care of an emergency. I always left my office door open, unless I was gone for the day. While I was away, the CEO made his visit. Coincidence? Yeah, right. I took care of the emergency in record time, but not quite quick enough. I bumped into the CEO and the head of the board, as they were leaving the IT Department. As I was approaching my office, I caught the Service Center manager opening my office door and turning on the lights in my office. I took a step back behind the last corner I had turned and the Service Center manager didn't know he'd been caught. Caught red-handed. Another conspiracy. That's right. They didn't want the CEO and/or the head of the Board of Directors to see what was hanging on my office wall. They sent me away, then shut my office door and turned off the lights so the CEO and the head of the Board wouldn't see the truth. Conspiracy, because it took more than one person to pull this off.

At first, I thought the Service Center manager wasn't smart enough to think of something like this on his own. I thought he was the type who could be coerced into conceiving it, and not realize it really wasn't his idea, but then I remembered the pure genius he exhibited when suggesting what I should do to get a raise and/or a promotion. Yes, he may have been smart enough to conceive this idea, but there's no way he would have done it on his own. No way. His manager had to be involved or know about it. The problem: He didn't know he got caught. He didn't know they got caught – until now. Two members of management involved in two conspiracies. Two conspiracies that I know about. Maybe there's more. Maybe when others read this story, there will be more to add to it. I'm betting if the whole truth came out, it would be enough to add another five or ten chapters to this book. That's the nice thing about self-publishing. I can add to it and re-publish it within days. The same for the paperback. A couple days work and it can also be changed.

I won't deny I'm a little eccentric. Maybe even a little paranoid. Maybe I'm a little crazy. You see, when you're rich and famous, and mentally a little off, you're usually considered eccentric. When you're a person of the lower income bracket, or of lesser means, you're usually considered crazy or insane.

I began wearing a Sport Jacket while at the office. I was doing it for a reason. I was hoping to get a reaction about it from the manager of the software division. On the first day I began wearing sport jackets, my manager was concerned I might be going on a job interview. He wasn't really concerned. He was just putting on a dog-and-pony-show for those standing nearby. Another one of those times when I wanted to stick my fingers down my throat to induce vomiting. How interesting. If my manager had a brain in his head, he would have known I wouldn't tell anyone in the company if I did have a job interview. The next response, about a week or two later, came from another manager. This was the manager I was targeting. He inquired about the jacket. I replied that, since I was going to be making six figures someday, I wanted to know what it felt like to dress accordingly. A picture is worth a thousand words, but a facial expression can be worth a million dollars, if you know how to read it. The look I received was no surprise. You know the look, don't you? It's the look that says: "You're nuts if you think you'll ever make six figures." I'm betting you've all seen that look at some point in your life. His facial expression said it all. Maybe this manager wasn't aware I had shared information at my last performance review indicating I should be making very close to six figures. At the very least, I should have been making double what I was making. If I were properly compared to some people who worked there during my time there, I should have been making triple what I was making. I wonder. I wander. I wonder. I wander.

Something unexpected happened before the re-org. A person who was there for over nine years quit and walked out the door. No notice. No warning. He walked out on the spot. Those who knew the truth weren't surprised. I wasn't surprised. This person made it clear to the head of HR there were multiple problems within the IT Department and with the way it was being managed and ran. What happened next? Nothing much. The company was only concerned with beating this man out of his unemployment. It's my opinion this person was discriminated against. Did the head of HR follow up and do anything? Did he do what should have been done? No, he did not. He should have talked to every employee in the entire department, based on what he was told. At the very least, he should have spoken to everyone in the networking division, but that did not happen. I suspect he did something and I also suspect I know what he did. I suspect another conspiracy took place. I'll expose it in the movie. In my opinion, the head of HR was just another chair-cover sucking up a nice big paycheck while waiting for retirement. Chair-Cover: Something best used to cover a chair in order to keep it free of dust or debris.

Some may have the opinion I should have went to HR, filed a grievance or complained to the VP. I truly don't feel it would have mattered. If you read the rest of this story, you might come to understand why I don't feel it would have mattered or done any good. You might even agree now.

Shortly after this fiasco, a position was posted for a Project Manager. Big pay and a proper title. Coincidence? Not at all. Would anyone be surprised to know if the person who quit and walked out the door just a couple months earlier had the title and pay grade of a Project Manager he wouldn't have left? Would anyone be surprised to know I couldn't apply for this position because I had already been told I would not receive the advancement I deserved? Would anyone be surprised to know I once did this job and had more experience doing it than anyone in the department at the time? Remember: I was told if I wanted to make more money to get a job down the hill in the software division. One of the questions on the Online Survey was about my manager creating a career path for me. It was his job. And he did not do his job. He never did anything remotely resembling the creation of a career path. Best place to work in Pa? No way, no how. Best place to be taken unfair advantage of. Best place to be discriminated against. Best place to be denied the advancement you really deserve. Best place to watch a group of managers make a bold-faced liar out of the CEO. I could go on, but that's enough for now.

I waited patiently for the re-org. I really had no choice. I wanted to see what crumbs I would be offered. At a division meeting everyone was told the Vice President was very involved and very supportive of this re-org. However, I later learned the VP was not involved enough, or at least not in my opinion. Or maybe there was some sort of a conspiracy going on. Could there have been a third conspiracy? I don't know for sure. My other reason for waiting was to see if things were finally going to change for me, and to see if this re-org would reflect statements made by the CEO and by my manager in my previous performance review. The re-org involved new titles and positions for almost everyone in the division. You had to apply for these positions via the job-posting system, be interviewed, and offered the position by HR. But in reality, the position is being offered by the manager, not HR. The manager decides who to offer the position to. I'm not sure who decides how much money to offer, but I suspect the manager has most of the input into it. So, the jobs were posted. At the time, I was the only person in the department with a Systems Engineer (MCSE) Certification. There were three positions which I was automatically qualified for, because they required having the MCSE certification as a condition of accepting the position or obtaining said certification within two years. I already had my MCSE certification, so naturally I figured it should be a slam-dunk for me, but seeing the jobs and descriptions didn't make any sense to me. I didn't see any descriptions relating to software deployment. It sounded like I was going to be squeezed into a position which needed filled, and my software deployment knowledge and experience was going to be part of the deal. How convenient. One might ask: "Who is watching the watchdogs?" Answer: Nobody. Who cares? Answer: Nobody.

In this re-org, all of the positions posted, including those in the service center, now required certifications. Let's compare that to the nursing structure. What happened here would be the equivalent of being certified as an RN, but working for the hourly pay of a CNA. Are there any nurses there with their RN credentials working for the hourly pay of a CNA? You don't have to answer that one. I already know the answer.

Hello, Mr. CEO. Are you listening? Apparently, a particular company email about your so-called "Pillars" wasn't read by my manager, or the Vice President I worked under. Maybe they didn't understand what it meant when it said "Better advancement opportunities for those with more years." You know the email I'm talking about, don't you? It's the one where you were bragging about all the great reasons to stay longer at this company. Maybe they did the old "dump and run" and forwarded your email to the entire department without reading it. Dump it on somebody else, get it off their plate, hot potato. Hot potato. Your email should have said: "Better advancement opportunities for those who are willing to bend over and be a suck-up and turn a blind eye to the truth and play the game the way management wants it to be played. If you're honest, efficient, and can save the company lots of money by way of efficiency or make the company millions utilizing your knowledge and experience, you need to stay at the bottom of the heap and be happy you have a job. We're the biggest employer in the area and we know it."

I was told getting certified would give me advancement. That didn't work. I was told to get a job down the hill. Who was supposed to create the career path which would get me a job down the hill? My manager, or the manager down the hill? Either way, that didn't work. I was told there would be a proper position created for me in the re-org. That didn't work. I was told about better advancement for those with more years. That didn't work. I was told this company is supposed to recruit and retain the best people and treat them well. That didn't work. I was told to be the squeaky wheel. That didn't work. I was told to show my manager the reasons why I deserved a raise and promotion. That didn't work. Tell me, Mr. CEO, what does work? How does it work? You don't have to answer the last question. I've already shown you how it works.

Maybe the problem was the mindset. Maybe the problem was the brains weren't moving as fast as the technology was. I was thinking my manager had the attitude it should take everyone as long to advance as it took him. But, when you look at all the various other positions created for all the various reasons, and sometimes political or idiotic reasons, one might find it hard to believe.

So, I waited patiently, thinking there had been a mistake. Maybe my position wasn't posted yet. I was thinking about applying for the network security team-leader position. It was a lead position and I already met the qualifications. And I had been in a team-leader role for over nine years.

Then, one afternoon, I was outside the building entrance. My manager came out the door and escorted me around the corner, out of public view. "Why haven't you applied for a position yet? You're holding up my re-org," he said. Let's break this down. If I'm the one holding up the re-org, wouldn't it indicate everyone else has applied for a position? It would to me. You see, this wasn't a re-org. It was a "control-org." It's an example of IT Management doing it their way. I responded I wasn't sure which one I wanted to apply for. My manager then said: "You should apply for the position of Data Storage Administrator." I explained how I wanted to apply for the Security Team Leader position, since I already had my MCSE certification, and I had aced the security portions with a 100% on all of the exams and I've been a team leader for over nine years at this company. I expected him to say something like: "You should apply for any position you feel qualified for or capable of doing," but that was not his response. His response was: "No, the Data Storage Administrator position is the one for you." I was preparing a response, which would have been a reminder about the information I shared at my last Performance Review pertaining to software deployment and the fact I already had my MCSE certification. Then my manager says: "Remember you once told me you could see yourself working on server setups some day or on the server team?" Yes, it was a true statement. Yes, I made that statement in my past. However, I made that statement many years ago and prior to getting my first big certification as a Systems Administrator. So, this is how a manager plans a career path? Please, Mr. CEO could you show us an example of how a career path is supposed to be planned? I sure can't figure it out. The only thing apparent here is this: My manager violated state labor laws by telling me what job I should apply for, and which one I shouldn't apply for. This is a free country and a person should be allowed to apply for any position within any company at any time. Can anyone understand why I was angry? What was the question on the Online Survey? Something about my manager planning a career path for me? Tell me, Mr. CEO - Did your manager plan a career path for you? Tell me, Mr. CEO, would you agree this manager just made a bold-faced liar out of you and your so-called "Pillars?"

My manager never planned a career path for me. He never even came close. That was another item in the Online Survey I gave a negative response to. If a career path would have ever been planned for me, I would have been a manager long ago. But, this was retaliation due to my honest feedback on the Online Survey. I will not apologize for it. I was honest. I did what I felt was proper. One problem was that the right people in the right places weren't aware of the job I was actually doing. I, as well as others, had concerns which management was not addressing, and concerns which have never been addressed, hence one of the reasons for my later departure. I had also shared over the years how I'd like to make a six-figure income someday, so why wasn't that position posted? Come on, Mr. Manager, I want to know why that position was never posted?

Many of you know how the game is played. They are in control. If you buck the system, the system will buck you. Going to HR would have only created more problems. As mentioned earlier, we're dealing with some sly foxes, and they'd have just found another way to get rid of me. Here are some questions I would like to have answered: Why was I the only person in the entire department with an MCSE certification, while three people came out of this re-org with titles and pay scales higher than me? Also note: They were given two whole years in which to get those certifications. Why was I in multiple team-leader roles for over nine years and now no longer a team leader? Why were four people made team leaders, when not a single one of them had any team-leader experience, to my knowledge? How interesting. Maybe the manager thought he was going to get away with discrimination. Isn't it discrimination when you are told to apply for a lesser position than three other open positions which you are qualified for which also offer higher compensation?

Do you see why I mentioned which position I wanted to apply for earlier? If I had received the correct answer from my manager, I could have applied for the job I wanted to apply for, even though the rate should have been another ten dollars an hour higher, in my case. But that wouldn't have worked for my manager. My manager knew if I was given the job I wanted to get, the software deployment would need to be done on overtime whenever it was needed. A statement I had made years ago, was being used as a way to control me, hold me down, hold me back, deny me what I truly deserved. Some might say I should be happy I received a promotion and a raise. That would be acceptable if it were a fair playing field, but it was not. It was just another example of discrimination on parade and management showing what your company is really about.

Three positions were posted requiring the MCSE certification. All three were filled by people who never even had a single Microsoft Certification in their life, and they were all given two years to obtain it. I already had my MCSE, but it didn't matter to my manager. One of the positions was filled by a person who not only didn't have any Microsoft certifications but was only employed there for about three years. What was it you said Mr. CEO? "Better advancement opportunities for those with more years." That was a lie. And don't give me a line of crap about the word "opportunity" because I didn't have the opportunity. I was told what job I had to apply for. I wasn't permitted to apply for the position I wanted to apply for.

Prior to the re-org, the previous security person left the company for another opportunity. I was interested in the position before the re-org was done. I was thinking about a future in security. I asked about how the position might be changed or affected by the re-org. I was told: "The security position will not be changing; it will be staying exactly the same." I also asked if there were any other changes coming relating to the security field and was told: "Nothing's going to change involving the security position in the re-org." More word games. Lies, lip-service, and bull-squat. I happened to know my manager had plans of creating a Lead Security position as part of the re-org. Not only had I heard this from another person in the department, but I had seen the re-org "road-map" on my manager's desk one day. I had arrived early for a meeting and there it was. When my manager arrived, the first thing he did was cover the chart. I suspect he left it there for a reason. I suspect my manager wanted me to see it. Once again, a display of an IT Manager flexing their muscles and walking around like a turkey strutting their stuff. To quote Aleister Crowley: "Do what thou wilt shall be the whole of the law."

Chapter 14

I later learned another manager in the department had denied a person a chance for advancement. This manager was the Director down the hill in the software division. A person wanted to apply for a management position in the other division, working under this Director, in the software division. He felt he was qualified. He'd been with the company for more than a few years. He spoke to the director of the software division who would be doing the hiring for the position and was told he needn't bother applying. He wasn't going to get the position and, if he didn't like it, he should consider leaving the company. I want it clearly understood I heard about this after the fact. I didn't witness it. It's what some would call "Hearsay." I believe this to be true. I believe others would also believe this to be true. Would it surprise you to learn this man was a black man? Would it matter? Would it surprise you to know this position was filled by someone who didn't currently work at the company? Would it surprise you to know the person I'm referring to here is the same black man mentioned earlier? As mentioned earlier, the manager who hired this black man was removed from his position. I'm wondering if there's ever been another black person hired in the department since my departure from the company. And what happened to the director who told this man to go pound dirt? He was promoted to Vice President. The rich get richer and the poor get told to go pound dirt.

I'm also wondering if this man might have given negative feedback on the Online Survey. I'd bet he did. Could it be the reason he was told not to apply for the position? Or, was the real reason they already knew who the position was going to be given to. Don't worry. The man got the hint. He left the company. The CEO's statement is ringing loud and clear: "Better advancement opportunities for those with more years." You see the problem here. When you're told not to apply for a job, you're being told you are not allowed to even try to advance or better yourself. And therefore, HR has no idea you want advancement. HR will never have it on the record you want advancement. This is what happens when IT Management runs their own HR Department. Either the CEO is a liar or multiple members of IT management made a liar out of him. Which is it? What came first? The chicken or the egg? If a CEO promised better advancement opportunities for those who were there longer, shouldn't it have been a policy at HR? If it was, then somebody was sleeping at the wheel and they were definitely sleeping at the wheel during the re-org. And what about the manager who told this employee to "go pound dirt?" What happened to him? As I said before: He got promoted to Vice-President. The foxes are watching the chickens in the pen; The problem is nobody watches them.

Down the hill. Get a job down the hill. Here's another observance I made while I worked at this company. During the nine-plus years I worked there, nobody from my division ever got a job down the hill. One man applied, but management decided to give it to somebody outside of the department, even though the position was initially posted for internal department candidates only. This person hinted he was going to complain to HR. There was a little management "Gang-bang" meeting with multiple managers present who convinced this employee not to go to HR. I wasn't there. I don't know what was said. I suspect it was another example of: "IT Management will do what they want, how they want, when they want, if they want, and for who they want. And if you don't like it, you should leave the company."

Here's another example of IT Management running their own HR department. The Clinical Manager retired. To my knowledge, his open position was never posted. He gave a two-week notice, did his two weeks, then left. Here's how it's supposed to work: A person gives a two-week notice. If they change their mind during those two weeks, they have the option to stay. But, their position isn't posted until, or unless they actually leave the company. This person's last day was on a Friday. The following Monday, it was announced who the new manager was for the clinical manager's position. To my knowledge, this position was never posted in the job-posting system.

Here's the problem. If someone had interest in advancement, HR would have no knowledge of it. If someone in the department, who'd been there longer, had interest in the position, HR would never know. I wonder if there's a loophole which allows something like this to happen. Since the position was never posted, nobody was allowed to apply for it if they did want it. I wonder if there were any employees who were there longer that may have had interest in this position? I wonder if the CEO was once again made a bold-faced liar. I wonder if the whole truth about this fiasco will ever come out.

I wonder if it's a coincidence that the director who hired this replacement manager and this new manager were both aware of the fact a manager with our primary software vendor expressed interest in having me do a presentation that year in Las Vegas, and did absolutely nothing about it. They didn't tell the VP, or Marketing, and they didn't tell the CEO. They didn't tell anyone. Don't ask, don't tell. That's how they played the game. On a side note here: If they did tell the VP, which I highly doubt considering the nature of how they ran things, then the VP did nothing. She'd be a good scapegoat, since she retired and no longer works there. But in my book, she retired a bold-faced liar and there's enough truth out there to prove it.

I mentioned earlier how this book might flush out one or more rats. I truly believe there was more than one rat. This is what happens when multiple conspiracies, which affected the futures of multiple employees, takes place. The only way to expose it is with the truth.

Chapter 15

During most of my time in the IT Department, I was overseeing the service team. I was responsible for assigning their work, knowing where they were and what they were working on, and being their technical go-to and first point of contact, if they needed assistance or guidance in the field. I didn't always know all of the answers, but I usually knew which direction to guide them, since I had a lot of knowledge about a majority of the systems and how they functioned. When I had to work on software deployment items, the service center manager would watch over the techs in my absence. Isn't that interesting? I wasn't being paid as a manager or a supervisor, but most of the time, a manager took over for me in my absence, including my vacation time.

Hello, Mr. CEO. Are you paying attention? I hope I'm not boring you. Wake up! Somebody made a fibber out of you, and you didn't even know it. Don't sweat it. It's normal. This kind of stuff goes on all over the country. You're not the first one. Somebody also made a fibber out of the former VP, or maybe she lied to everyone. You figure it out. I no longer care. I used to care, but after you've been lied to and discriminated against enough, you reach a point where you no longer care. If somebody else would have cared, I, along with some others, might still be there. Maybe your company would still exist, as its own entity.

If I would have been the Vice-President, I can promise you I would have been bird-dogging every single part of this Online Survey fiasco to find out what the problems were, what the truth was, why it happened, what needed fixed, was it fixed and, most importantly, was it fixed properly? And I would have been meeting with every single hourly employee within the department one-on-one to insure it was properly addressed, regardless of how much time it would have taken. But that's just how I would have done things. That's what I would have done, or would do, if I were the Vice-President. I would consider it a personal short-coming in my own performance as a leader if there was so much wrong. Maybe that's why I didn't make it that far up the ladder. I knew the Vice-President didn't really care. I don't sugar-coat things, I don't fluff it under the carpet, and I don't do the old "dump-and-run." I wouldn't be a Lemming. I wouldn't have hidden out in a glass castle waiting for it to blow over. There are some who might say this is a character flaw. I won't apologize for it. My creator made me this way for a reason.

If any manager had any type of a problem with you, forget the idea of proper or fair advancement, it would not happen. And if you didn't like it, or had a complaint, you would be encouraged to leave. And if you were tired of hitting brick walls, do not complain or be honest about it on the Online Survey. That will be a big waste of your time, and it might be used against you. It was most definitely used against me, as well as others. These surveys are sometimes done so a company can look good on paper. I remember a communication giving congratulations to everyone in this company for helping the company be recognized as one of the best places to work. It was based on feed-back from the Online Survey. I wonder if anybody knows the survey results were tainted? When management changed the survey to being done by sections, instead of the entire department, as it was when they received such a large amount of negative feedback, they tainted the survey. Did they think the average person would want to be honest and open about their opinions in the following survey? I don't know what they thought, but I know multiple people didn't agree with it being done that way. Doing it that way allowed them to look at their feedback by smaller groups and sections. Then, they would be able to try to figure out who the individuals were who had a complaint or provided negative feedback. The saddest part of this whole story is if they really cared, they wouldn't have received such an enormous amount of negative feedback to begin with.

This company allows the problem to fix the problem. The problem was management. But management refused to accept they needed to change. They felt fixing the employees or getting certain employees to leave was the answer. I don't think it ever occurred to any of them they might be wrong. Absolute power corrupts absolutely. Prior to that change being made I heard some mention they were not going to complete another one of those surveys, because they felt nothing was going to change and because they didn't feel things had been addressed properly. Some said they'd fill it out with answers that were all very negative or check the box that said: "Strongly Disagree" because they knew nothing was going to change and they wanted to send another message. Where is it written a person deserves respect just because of their title or position? Shouldn't respect be earned, not deserved?

Various companies spend millions of dollars on Marketing and bragging about being a "Great Place" to work. For some companies, it's just a scam. Part of the problem is the system. These surveys aren't regulated. You pay the survey company a fee, employees take the survey, and then the company can do whatever it wants with the survey data. There are even some companies who don't have the guts to hear from all of their employees for a survey. They select a group of employees to take the survey. Then, they try to claim this group is a fair representation of the entire company. I wonder how that scam works? I feel it is a scam. Is this done to save money? Is it done so the company only pays for a hundred surveys as opposed to five thousand? I don't think this is proper. There needs to be regulations put in place to ensure these surveys are a true representation of all employees who work for a company.

The hospital I worked at is now pulling this scam. I say scam, because I don't believe the survey results are accurate. I suspect they decide a year in advance who will take the survey, and then treat those employees with all kinds of kindness until the survey results are in. I also suspect the idea may have come from some of the managers who were involved in the conspiracy which took place when I worked there. If a company is going to brag about being a "Great Place" to work, it should be a result of survey answers given by every single employee in the company. It should not include answers or results from any sub-contracted company. There lies another problem. Some hospitals (and other companies) have hundreds of employees who are employed by another company. They call them things like "business partners" or "partners in service" or "partners in success." The reality is they are not company employees. They are a business expense. They are a tax write-off. That's what they really are. I'm not saying their contribution isn't helpful or important, but their survey results should not be part of the mix when it comes to claiming a title of "Great Places." Those employees should take a survey paid for by the company they work for. It should not be combined with the company they sub-contract from and it should have nothing to do with the location they work at. Their answers should reflect the company who signs their paychecks, not the location where they work. They are not employees of the company at the location where they work.

Now, I'm going to play a word game. I'm going to share some words I've heard over the years. I'm also going to share some information many thought had been shoved under the carpet. Welcome to the grand opening of Pandora's Box. Why did these things happen? Am I the only one? I'm not the only one. People who find it so easy to operate in this way have the opinion they can get away with it because nobody will say anything. They think the need for a future personal reference will give them the edge if an employee whom they treated unfairly decides to move on. They figure fear will be a good motivator to keep somebody in check, to hold them down and to hold them back or to keep them around as long as they were willing to work for less compensation than others. It might just work if the person in question is going to be dependent on them, but what they fail to realize is some people can work in different fields and do different things. They also might be thinking some will just go out the door with their tail between their legs, never to be heard from again. But there's also another type of person. I'm the other type of person. You can kick a dog and beat him. He may put up with it for a while. He might not even show you his teeth while you abuse him. He might disappear, never to be seen or heard from again. Some dogs might just get up one day and decide to bite back.

Hello again, Mr. CEO. I want to share why this happened. Your company has what's known as an unwritten "Don't ask, don't tell" Policy. Here's an example: You and Marketing spend all kinds of time, effort, and energy spouting off about how great your company is to work for. Emails, speeches, blah-blah-blah. They're all just tall tales to sucker people into staying longer. Better opportunities, you're a partner here, blah-blah-blah. The truth is far from it. Have you or anyone in the company ever told anyone what to do if they were lied to or discriminated against? Answer: No. Reason: You live in a constant state of delusion and denial believing everything is just fine. Once you get to the management level, the rules change to: "I'm getting my nice salary and that's all that really matters. If the peons have a problem, we can get more peons. There are plenty of them out there."

There are many who might say: "This manager has always been nice to me, I've never had a problem with our department's managers, or management. I've never had a problem with any manager." It may well be the case for some people. Sometimes the truth takes a while to come out. The scandal at Penn State might be a good example of the truth taking a while to come out. Remember, there were even a few serial-killers who were well-liked by somebody. Some were well-liked by everyone who met them. I remember a little joke from the past: "You can make hoagies all of your life, and be the best hoagie-maker in town, but if you rob one bank, do you think they'll call you a hoagie-maker?" Also remember, I'm not the only one who had some bad experiences with some of these managers. I'm just the first one to come forward and go public. Albert Einstein once said: "If you want to fool the world, tell the truth."

Chapter 16

Tell us, Mr. CEO: How did it work when you came up through the ranks? I'd really like to know. How did you become CEO? Do you know the whole story? Do you know the real truth? I don't think you do. You are about to have a rude awakening. The whole truth. I'm going to let you in on another one of my secrets and tell you how you became CEO.

I was involved in a little private tour of a nearby shopping center. The tour happened early in the morning. The former CEO had apparently arranged a purchase of this property without the consent or knowledge of the Board. He also arranged for the purchase of a nearby high-rise, with the intention of tearing it down and building the new hospital at this location. There were about a dozen people at this private little tour. Four or five of them were managers. My manager was there. The idea was to plan for networking, phone systems, and all of the other needed items. We were told this property had been purchased from the city. Apparently these purchases were being arranged or done through some "shadow company" know as "The Bread Box" or "The Bread Basket" or a name similar to one of those just mentioned. I don't know who actually oversaw this shadow company, nor do I care. I don't know if it's 100% true, but I believe it is. We were told not to wear any clothing which would identify who we worked for. We were told not to have our hang-tags hanging on the mirrors of our vehicles.

These tags had the name of the hospital on them. This was a secret operation. I knew there was something smelly in Denmark. Something very smelly, indeed.

Later that same morning after returning to my office, I sent an anonymous letter to the Board of Directors via the internal company mail system. I even wrote the date and the time on the letter. I also sent copies to multiple others. I will not disclose who they are or why I chose these particular individuals to receive a copy. The letter stated the facts about the secret tour. It asked why it was being kept a secret? It asked the Board if they were aware their CEO might be doing something without their consent or knowledge.

A couple days later, I had a talk with my manager. I knew the letters I sent would have been received by this time. I'm sure the one I sent to the board was received. I shared my concerns about this little tour with my manager. I explained I would have expected some kind of blessing from one of the sisters, because there were some Nuns affiliated with this hospital, or a statement in the local press about the recently acquired plaza. I also wondered why the other property wasn't mentioned publicly. Everyone was under the impression the new hospital building was going to be built at the existing location as an expansion and the existing building was going to be added on to. If it's going to be built at a different location, why the big secret? That would have been front-page news. We're talking about a company that spends huge amounts of money on Marketing. They do television ads, full-page newspaper ads, and radio ads. They spend lots of money to make sure everyone knows who they are, and how great they are. They jump into the spotlight at every chance they get. A headliner story, but this headline was never printed. Once again, I got the look. Do you remember the look? The million-dollar look? The one where the facial expression says: "You're totally bonkers. You're crazy. You're nuts." I know the look. I've seen it more times than I can recall. This time I was getting the look from my manager. A person with the title of Director. Another chair-cover. I have quite a collection of chair-covers and the collection is getting bigger and bigger. I knew I hadn't been taken seriously, or my manager was afraid to question anyone about my concerns.

Did the board ever receive my letter? I don't know. How did they really find out? I don't know. Did they receive the letter, keep it a secret, then find out the truth through other means or did they find out through one of the others whom I sent the letter to? I don't know. Would the Board of Directors ever admit they learned about this fiasco via an anonymous letter? I don't know. But I can tell you what I do know. I know a couple days after I sent the anonymous letters out, there was a front-page story in the morning paper. A headliner. The headline read: "Hospital CEO Resigns!" Coincidence? Big coincidence. Huge coincidence. Shortly afterwards, there was another front-page story announcing the newly appointed CEO. Was my manager responsible for the board finding out? If he was, I certainly didn't get the recognition for it. If he was, he took all the credit. But remember, It was I who suspected it first. It was I who took action first. Don't ask, don't tell.

Some may think this plaza story is ridiculous. It's not. It's true. There's more than one person out there who knows the truth. The former CEO didn't make these arrangements without some kind of written or verbal agreement from one or more members of the local city council, or possibly county administration knowing about it or somehow being in the loop. The truth is out there somewhere. I know it is. Something this big has to have some kind of a trail, and I believe it's on the record somewhere. If it's not on the record, it's in someone's memory.

Hello again, Mr. "Newly Appointed" CEO. Were you paying close attention earlier when asked how you came up through the ranks? I just told you how. You didn't know the whole story, did you? I'm thinking the above information will probably be denied, or not believed in its entirety. I'm not able to prove any of it, and I won't disclose how many letters were sent. Nor will I disclose who they were sent to, other than the one labeled: Board of Directors. But, you must admit, it surely seems like one heck of a coincidence. Is it true or false? It's not important. You would probably have been the next logical choice for CEO regardless of the circumstances which got you there. But, would you have made CEO in your lifetime at this company, if the previous CEO wouldn't have screwed up? I don't think so. You've done quite well for yourself, Mr. CEO. I seem to recall you are a board member of a very large worldwide organization. Would it have happened if you weren't the CEO? I wonder. I wander. I wonder. I wander. I'm also curious to know if you stayed an extra week in your previous position prior to moving into the position of CEO.

If anyone decides to take me seriously about the above matter, I'm sure the proof is out there somewhere. I'm sure someone within the city or county ranks knew about this. The facts listed above are not the utterances of a delusional or schizophrenic person. The truth is there if someone were to search for it. Those who were involved at the city and/or county level have kept it a secret. Now, it's no longer a secret, because I've exposed it.

I once read an article about the cost of keeping employees who perform poorly. Has anyone ever looked at the cost of keeping managers who perform poorly? How much employee turnover can be attributed to an improper management structure? How much employee turnover can be attributed to poor management practices, methods, and tactics? This would be very hard to find out. Who should do it? How should it be done? There needs to be a system of checks and balances in place, and at your company - there most certainly isn't.

How dare your company send me a letter asking for feedback about my experiences working there after I left and was no longer employed there? How dare you? Why didn't you ever send me such a letter while I worked there? In the nine-plus years I worked there, nobody cared to ask. The only thing which came close to asking was the Online Survey. And when we answered it honestly, we were black-balled by this company. I hope by now you realize, Mr. CEO, I could have most certainly brought and won a discrimination suit against you. By your own words under the so-called "Pillars" I was discriminated against. I chose not to pursue a discrimination suit. I know what the outcome would have been. The liars would keep lying and I'd get nothing or, I'd get offered much less than I should have and been and forced to sign a non-disclosure agreement. Either way, the truth would have been buried. This way, the truth comes out.

I did some research and basic math. This information is based on my experience. I don't have the coveted four-year degree which your company seems to place such great importance on. My math might be skewed. Two-year college addition, subtraction, and division might be different than those taught at the four-year college level. It's my opinion at least ten people (that's ten people at a minimum) left the company because of what I'm sharing about in this story. Ten times 30 years each = 300 years of service. I'm basing this on the employee staying thirty years, since you brag about how much better it is to stay longer. Now, let's do two directors, three managers and one Vice President. That's a total of six, I think. Yup, six it is. Sorry, it took me a while to figure it out. Not having a four-year degree takes me a little longer to cipher things out. It took me a while to apply something you can't get with a four-year degree: Common sense. I can add these numbers on my fingers. One two three four five six. Looks like six. Let's get back to the facts. Let's say this group is going to stay for thirty years each. That's 180 years of service. Wow! Do you see what I see? Did I do the math properly? It appears ten hourly employees would give more to the company than six managers. If you fired the ten hourly employees, could these six managers do their job? Could six people do the work of ten? So, removing six problems to keep ten solutions makes sense to me. But, then again, I am an "out of the box" thinker, so there's really no way my common-sense approach would be accepted as such. Remember: I'm not eccentric, I'm crazy. I don't fall into the proper income category to be considered eccentric. Forget I mentioned it. Down boy. Bad dog. Go lay down and play dead, Rover. Roll over and hope for a belly-rub. Pray for a bone tossed down from a throne.

That's 300 years of lost service, for ten employees. The company would have only lost 180 years of service by eliminating six managers. I wonder if anyone else ever looked at it that way? I wonder if the Board of Directors or the CEO would be brave enough to contact every former employee who left the department while I was there, and since

I left, to find out how much of this is really true? Would the CEO or the Board of Directors be brave enough to poll (and give them total anonymity) all of the current employees for the truth? The problem is some may choose to keep things under their belt due to fear of retaliation or a bad employment reference. I'm not saying they would be wrong for doing just that. They've all seen these sly foxes in action. Most of them (the hourly employees, not members of management) would probably say they were just wanting a change, or a better opportunity appeared. But there might be a few who might tell you a whole lot more if they were promised anonymity. It's a gray area. I wonder how many years of lost service might have occurred in other departments? I talked to a few people over the years and you'd be very surprised to know what I've heard from various employees in other departments. But, I won't break their confidentiality. They deserve better and they also deserve a lot better than what they've been getting.

Chapter 17

To smoke or not to smoke. That is the question. Smoking is legal. There's no law against it. Why are hospitals getting away with discrimination where smokers are concerned? Multiple hospitals nationwide are denying employment because of smoking. I'm wondering when somebody is going to put their foot down. No company in this country should be able to deny employment to someone because they smoke cigarettes. Many of them would probably say it relates to being self-insured and helps keep costs down. If that's the reason, then a smoker should just pay a higher rate, as they would with any other insurance company. Maybe certain hospitals would say it offends their customers or patients. Get over it. With the advances made in breath fresheners and air-fresheners, they wouldn't know an employee was a smoker.

Why not ask the patient before they're admitted? If it bothers them, make sure they're attended to by non-smokers. That's almost how it worked in the old days, back when you could smoke as a patient in your hospital bed. When a patient was admitted, they were asked if they preferred a smoking or non-smoking room. I don't see the big problem. I do see the bigger problem: Discrimination.

Your customers are going to smell a smoker when they visit the mall, the grocery store, or any number of places visited by the public. What's next? Are you going to deny a visitor the right to set foot on your property because they smoke? These discriminatory practices are going on nationwide, and nobody seems to want to call it what it really is: Discrimination. Maybe someday a person will somehow prove they were denied employment or fired for being a smoker. Maybe said person will get a good law firm and sue for millions. Maybe that's what it will take. But the reality is the Board of Labor knows about this. They know it goes on in multiple states and in multiple companies and they're playing the good 'ole "Don't ask, don't tell" game. Some hospitals all but tell you they won't hire you if you're a smoker, or you must quit within so many days of being hired as a condition of your employment there.

I recall a funny incident. The CEO was putting on a presentation about the upcoming building expansion. Many felt the Board of Directors had no business taking the company into so much debt. Many felt the project was too aggressive. I recall seeing a picture of a boat full of people and being told a story about rowing the boat a little harder, or something along those lines. Multiple employees joked about this when things were hectic. They'd say: "Just row the boat a little harder." I don't recall seeing any members of management in the boat doing any of the rowing. I don't recall seeing anyone wearing a suit or a tie. Maybe they were all busy attending meetings or reading and sending emails that day. Maybe it was one of the lifeboats from the Titanic and they missed boarding the Titanic on that particular day. I must confess my vision isn't the best. I was wearing reading glasses and might not have seen the boat clearly.

I always had the opinion this company was destined to fail. There wasn't enough common sense being used. There were some conflicts of interest within this company, in my opinion. Multiple members of the board were business owners who did business with the company. In my opinion, this should never happen, except under certain types of controlled circumstances. I'm wondering if this happens nationwide? Does this happen at other hospitals? Does it happen at other companies? I always felt this was not proper. It's only my opinion it was a conflict of interest. I decided not to share any of those examples. I'm saving them for the movie.

Some would say the company didn't fail. I would say they did. They got in over their head and had to have help to continue as the entity they had always claimed to be. They could have remained autonomous and they could have remained in business, but they would have had to make serious cuts in various areas. One of those areas might have been the amount they gave back to the community. But it's my opinion if this company had continued on in the same way it had been doing in the past, it most definitely would have ended up in trouble.

What do you do when your company is heading down the tubes and you're looking for a partner or looking to form an alliance with a bigger company?

You get marketing on the job. You start putting out propaganda to lead the public into thinking this was something you were hoping for, and looking for, all along. You might even go so far as to brag about how well you're doing and how you have tens of millions in revenues, blah-blah-blah. Do you really think the person on the street is stupid enough to believe you? If you do, maybe you are just as eccentric as I am crazy. It doesn't matter if you have a billion dollars in yearly revenue, if your expenses are one penny over a billion dollars, you lost money. You did not make a profit. You didn't even break even. I would like to cipher this out for you, but I don't have a four-year degree and I don't have enough fingers and toes to count that many digits.

Chapter 18

I seem to recall some propaganda about this hospital being such great financial stewards. Here's a couple of examples of how some of their money was spent.

It was decided coffee might not be supplied to the IT employees and a group was formed to address this issue. The group consisted of five or six hourly employees and even a manager. I was asked to be on the committee. I was a big coffee drinker. I won't tell you how many meetings we held, nor will I tell you how long it went on. In the end, it was decided the department would continue furnishing coffee, since a lot of it was consumed by various others who came there to use the training rooms. What do you think? Is this a good example of being a great financial steward?

Another example would be my departure. About a month after I left the company, I was contracted to come back and share some knowledge about software deployment. Apparently, my former manager wanted to make some kind of an impression, or send me a message. I shared a small bit of knowledge about software deployment. There were three people present at this little meeting. One was the team leader I was forced to work under, due to my manager discriminating against me. The other person was a member of the Data Storage team I worked on. The other person was the Project Manager who held the position I wasn't allowed to apply for, because I was told if I wanted a raise to get a job down the hill. Near the end of this little dog-and-pony show, my former manager appeared to say hello and ask how things were going. Now for the good part: What I showed them could have been learned by any one of them by launching one piece of software and clicking on the word "Help." What I shared with them was no secret, nor was it based on my years of deployment experience. The average tenth-grader could have learned it without any help, training, or assistance. The problem is: There's never a tenth-grader around when you need one. One hundred dollars an hour. That's what this company paid out in order to learn what could have been learned within thirty minutes of clicking "Help." What I showed them was a small piece of the software deployment puzzle. I won't tell you how long I was there. If I was there ten minutes, it was a major waste of company resources. Of course, you all know the reason for this fiasco. It was to let me know I would not be returning there to do consulting work. What do you think? Is this a good example of being a great financial steward? I could show you many more, but I'm saving them for the movie.

Prior to my departure, the economy was taking a turn for the worse. In one of our staff meetings, the VP started the meeting by mentioning multiple companies who were either laying off employees or closing their doors. "It's getting really bad out there," she said. Did she really think the employees didn't know what was going on with the economy?

Was she really that stupid? I'm not sure. I think it was her way of saying: "You could be next." I'm wondering if this type of statement, or words to that effect, were shared by other managers or directors at other staff meetings? I'm wondering if the VP ever thought about the idea that, if there was downsizing, it would and should most definitely start at the management level, since there were a few managers who couldn't possibly do the job of any one of their subordinates? I'm also wondering if I'm the only one who ever felt the company had twenty-five percent more managers than it needed? I wonder. I wander. I wonder. I wander.

My manager had a saying. He used to say it quite often: "Choose your battles." The sad reality is there shouldn't be battles to choose from. If the goal is to do things properly, the so-called battles should be few and far between. Too bad my manager forgot to tell me when to choose my battles. I chose now. Years later. But this is not a battle. The war is long over. I just wanted to set the record straight. I also want others to be aware the truth is now out. I'm now going to share some of the battles I didn't choose. There's also some examples of this great financial stewardship which was bragged about by the CEO of this company.

A manager in the IT Department was using her computer for coupon clipping. The PC got so corrupted it had to have the operating system re-installed and all of her documents and information restored from backups. This happened twice within ninety days. I wonder how many hourly employees ever did such a thing. What was the outcome? Were they written-up? Does it surprise anyone a manager has time to look for good deals on the company computer while sucking-up a management salary? But there was no money in the budget for me to get a raise, or proper advancement. And where is this manager now? I heard a rumor she got a better paying management position in another department. I don't know if it's true, but that's what I heard. I didn't choose to fight this battle, but I did make sure my manager was aware of it. I also made a comment on the Online Survey about discipline not being fairly and/or properly administered. I suspect some hourly employees were written up for merely visiting sites which weren't allowed by their department's policy. I wonder if any were fired for this? If so, how many infractions did it take? You see, if this was made public when it happened, there's a good chance a few people may have had grounds for a discrimination lawsuit. Isn't it discriminatory to punish one person, but not another for the same violation?

While standing in the lunch line one day a doctor was complaining to the cashier he should get his meals for free. I was angered by this. Why didn't the doctor negotiate it into his employment contract? What a jerk. I felt sorry for the cashier. She was a very nice person who was making just over minimum wage. She was a person who was always friendly and greeted everyone with a smile. I also felt sorry for the doctor. I didn't realize doctors couldn't afford to buy their own lunch. I didn't choose to fight this battle. I chose to inform my manager. Now, I will tell you what would have happened if I were the manager being told about this. I would have informed somebody. If I would have been CEO when such an idiotic statement was made, I would have personally required the doctor give an apology that very same day. It didn't align with the four-letter program the company was always bragging about. Don't get the wrong idea, I have the utmost respect for doctors. I don't have the utmost respect for jerks. I'm wondering if my manager reported this incident to anyone? I'm betting the answer is no.

Software licensing. Now here's a big one. I chose not to fight this battle. When the company went live on a new system, I informed my manager Microsoft SQL CALS (Client Access Licenses) needed to be purchased for every PC accessing the clinical system. The answer came back a day later. According to the vendor, an SQL CAL wasn't needed because an interface account on the server was doing the inputting, appending, or changing the data. I suggested Microsoft be contacted for clarification. My manager replied: "No, we're not going to contact Microsoft. I already know what their answer will be." If he already knew the answer, then he was basically saying: "Up yours, Microsoft. I don't have to buy your licenses, even though a Microsoft Certified Professional told me I should." I know I was right. Every single Microsoft Certification exam I've ever taken had questions about SQL CALS and when they must be purchased. Nobody wanted to hear what I had to say. You remember me? I'm the only person in the department who was certified by Microsoft at the time. I'm wondering if any of the designers of this system were Microsoft Certified. Don't ask, don't tell. Since the vendor said we didn't need SQL CALS, we got our fall guy. Interpretation: When it hits the fan we'll blame the vendor. This is what happens when you do it fast and not right. Had the project been properly planned, there would have been enough money to buy the licenses. That's what it was really about. The money. I must clarify I did not hear this from the vendor. I was told by my manager, who informed me he was told by the Clinical Manager, who apparently was in contact with the vendor about this subject. I must clarify this because my manager had a track record of lying to me. It's possible the vendor was never in the loop concerning the subject at hand.

Now, for the big picture. What if other hospitals were told by this vendor they didn't need SQL CALS for this system? What if I am 100% correct, and they are all wrong? I know SQL licenses were needed for this system. This could mean Microsoft might be owed over 500 million in licensing fees, give or take a 100 million. Is this system used in other countries worldwide? If so, Microsoft could be owed over a billion dollars total in licensing fees. That would also mean all of these hospitals might have a serious problem. If I am correct, I wonder who would be held responsible for paying for all of these licensing fees? I can't speak for any other hospital, but at the one I worked at, I feel they are responsible. They are responsible because they were told they needed to purchase these licenses by a Microsoft Certified Professional, but they chose to ignore the professional. Who knows, maybe they'll all get a free pass. I wonder if Microsoft knows they might be owed over half a billion. They've already made lots of money, so maybe they wouldn't care. Come on, laugh! That was supposed to be funny.

What about the competition? What if competitors lost business to this vendor? Is it possible some hospitals chose this software vendor because they were under the impression they wouldn't need to purchase SQL licenses? I don't know. I do know if I owned a company which lost market share because of this, I would definitely be suing somebody to recoup my losses. It would be the proper thing to do for the company and for the shareholders.

What about companies which have nothing to do with healthcare? What if the information in this book is true? Here's why there needs to be a thorough investigation and audit by various software companies who do business with healthcare. If I owned a company and found out there were companies who didn't buy these licenses, and weren't somehow held accountable, would I be entitled to a refund or a rebate? Do you see the big picture? If a hospital was supposed to spend a half a million for SQL CALS, but didn't, what about the half a million I spent buying them? Once again, a private company has shareholders. Wouldn't their returns be reduced due to the amount spent on software licensing? I can promise you, if I owned a company and had knowledge of something along these lines, I'd be demanding a refund from my software vendor. I'd be screaming and crying: No fair, foul, not right, not fair, shouldn't be allowed.

While we're on the subject of software compliancy, what about the law? In most states, it's a felony to commit software piracy. I saw a movie once where someone mailed letters and was charged a felony for each letter mailed. If there were two thousand computers in question, did I witness two thousand individual felonies? The system had a major upgrade which was performed prior to my departure. Does this mean I witnessed a total of four thousand felonies?

While we're on the subject of licensing, here's another example of abuse of power. We installed software at the hospital where I worked. We also installed software at other hospitals where we subbed our Techs to their companies. Those companies bought their own licenses. We would install the software. Things were tracked well and I believe these other hospitals were software-compliant, from a licensing perspective - Until now. A small project came up at one of these hospitals and they needed dozens of a certain kind of license. Our company had lots of these which were no longer in use, so my manager decided it was ok to just give these licenses to this other hospital. I personally witnessed this manager tell our IT Software Compliancy person (This was just one of the hats this person also wore) not to be wining about buying licenses because we had hundreds of them in our possession. Did I just witness a felony, or multiple felonies being committed?

Here's what really happened. Now, two hospitals have committed a form of software piracy. The other hospital (the customer) didn't even know it. They weren't even aware of it. They didn't have anyone in their company responsible for software compliancy. If they did, I don't believe this person was aware of what happened. Software was installed on computers at their company that was not purchased by their company. That's violation number one. Software licensing was transferred from the company I worked at to their company. That's violation number two. I'll tell you why. A tenth grader could figure this one out. Once again, there's never a tenth grader around when you need one. When you install a piece of software on any computer, there is a screen in which, or on which, you must accept the software company's terms of use. One of those terms of use statements clearly states: "This software is not to have ownership transferred without the express written permission of the company." Or, it might say: "Your company has Non-Transferable rights to install and use this software on one device Owned and Operated at purchasing company." According to my count, my manager has now committed software piracy at two different companies. Another battle I chose not to fight. How many others were there? I'll keep that answer to myself. A little more juice for the movie.

We did an upgrade to active directory while I was there. Before going to active directory, we had to upgrade our email system. This was a multi-tiered migration because our email system was two, or maybe more, versions behind the current system. Here's a short explanation of how email is licensed when running Microsoft Exchange. You have to buy a license for each mailbox. When you upgrade, you have to buy licenses for every mailbox you have, based on the version you are upgrading to. We did a multi-tiered upgrade. I can't recall if we migrated through two versions or more. To my knowledge, we bought the licenses for the final version we migrated to, but I don't believe we bought the licenses for the version, or versions, in between. Maybe Microsoft has a special pass for this, allowing you to upgrade to the latest and greatest without buying the versions you migrated past, but as a Microsoft Certified Professional, I never heard of or encountered this special "free pass" license which was used. Did I bring this to my manager's attention? No, I did not. Once shame on you, twice shame on me. He didn't listen to me the first time I told him we needed to buy licenses, so there was no reason for me to believe he'd listen to me any time afterwards. I adopted the unwritten policy which was continuously shown to me by IT Management: Don't ask, don't tell.

I'm not sure about the law here, but in most states, software piracy is a felony. Would it be a felony for every single license or would they just add up multiple years of conviction time for multiple felonies? I bring this up because a person was charged with a crime while I worked there. The crime didn't happen at the company. It had nothing to do with the company. But - company policy required this person to be terminated. If the person was cleared of the crime and found innocent, he (or she) could re-apply for a position in the company but was not promised getting their former job or position re-instated. This is very strange. What if I had made a criminal accusation towards a member of management? Would they have been terminated? If a man robs a bank, but never gets caught, is he a felon?

Different strokes for different folks. Here's another battle I chose not to fight. I go to fix a laptop. High Priority. Urgent. It's a doctor. Must have it quick. You don't want to risk impacting patient care. What was wrong with the laptop? It was polluted with spy-ware. It got there via multiple porn sights the good doctor had been visiting. It had to be the doctor because this device was one which had been provided specifically for this doctor, or the doctor ignored the "Portable Device User Agreement" he signed and allowed someone else to use the laptop. One of the requirements was for a user-agreement contract to be signed stating no other person would use the device. Also note: I understand in some medical areas of expertise, research could be confused with questionable graphics, etc. In this case, this physicians specialty had absolutely nothing to do in any way, shape, or form with what I discovered on his laptop. I provided the porn list and the other evidence to my manager. Do I need to tell you what happened afterwards? Obviously, nothing.

I was still overseeing the service team when one of the techs was investigating a strange problem on a PC. He mentioned to our manager he suspected porn as the culprit. The manager wasted no time responding. His response: "If it is, I'll call the police." I'm very confused. Mr. Manager didn't call the police when I had shown him absolute proof of porn surfing in the past on a Doctor's laptop, but he was ready to call the police when porn was the suspected culprit on the computer of an hourly employee. Can you see why I didn't choose this battle? Too bad none of the internal company training I had during my time there said I was supposed to call the cops if I saw the law broken, or a felony committed. I think only managers were allowed to call the cops.

Maybe I was supposed to call Marketing? No, not marketing. I was only supposed to direct people to marketing if they needed a comment, like a media reporter. I wasn't allowed to comment, or be interviewed by the media about anything involving this company, unless it was approved by marketing. So, if a reporter were to ask me if I ever witnessed a felony being committed at this company, I would say: No comment. You need to contact marketing to get permission for me to answer that question. That would be the proper way. They are in control.

I kept a loose tab on various activities relating to this subject. I won't tell you how many times I found questionable activity on computers and laptops of multiple doctors, managers, supervisors, or hourly employees. I'll save it for the movie. I'm going to present it the way your company taught me to do it. I'll do it if I want, when I want, how I want, and for who I want. Guess who's wearing a nice big crap-eating grin now?

I remember a big lawsuit which was avoided by this hospital. The judge refused to hear the case. The company lawyer (we'll call him Jake) was given major kudos for a job well done. The VP made it very clear to everyone at the next staff meeting how important this accomplishment was. "We couldn't have done it without Jake," she said.

Can Lawyers read? It seems Mr. Lawyer had a problem with his laptop one day. I assigned a tech and followed up personally for a status report. The laptop had some software installed on it which was not installed, or permitted, per the company policy. It was not installed by one of our techs. It was installed by Mr. Lawyer. It was gaming software for children. Once the tech removed the gaming software, the laptop worked fine. I'm figuring maybe Mr. Lawyer didn't read the agreement he signed prior to receiving his laptop. Maybe he missed the part stating he was the only one who was supposed to be using the laptop. I'm not saying he allowed a child to use his laptop, maybe he was the one playing children's games on this device. I don't know for sure. Maybe he missed the statement informing him software was not allowed to be installed, unless approved and installed via the IT Department. I thought it was very strange to learn a lawyer would have signed an agreement which he hadn't fully read and/or understood. Was Mr. Manager made aware of this fact? Yes, he was. Shortly after the tech completed the repair, Mr. Manager showed up and I provided him with the details about what caused the problem. Can anyone guess what happened next? I wonder how many hourly employees were written up or fired for doing similar things on their devices? Isn't this an example of discrimination? It is in my book. No doubt about it.

I'm wondering what might have happened if I had chosen this battle? I'm also wondering what might have happened if I sued this company for discrimination concerning the multiple ways I was discriminated against? Would the lawyer have had to step down, since he would be getting called as a witness? Would the lawyer have lied to the judge? Would a judge believe the word of two hourly employees or would the judge believe the lawyer? I'm sure my manager would have lied. No doubt about it. He's lied to me multiple times. Could your company have won a discrimination suit without Jake? Wouldn't it have been a major embarrassment to have it known to the public your own lawyer, who saved you millions in a previous suit, would have to step aside and be called as a witness in a discrimination suit involving your company?

Some might say it would be a stretch for this to happen, but would it? Wouldn't it be considered "Fruit from the poisonous tree?" One of my comments was about discipline not being fairly or properly administered. I believe I would have been well within my rights to demand this lawyer step down and be called as a witness.

There were many other battles I chose not to fight. More than the average person would expect. Some are funny, some are serious, some are idiotic, some are very sad. I decided they should be saved for the movie.

Chapter 19

The Mission Statement. Employees were required to memorize the Mission Statement and carry a miniature copy of it in the little pouch behind their employee badges. Managers were required to do the same. After I left the company, and was no longer an employee there, I returned and had a quick little chat with my former manager. I shared some personal and private information with him. The Mission Statement said something about extending God's healing something or other blah-blah-blah. I can assure you on that day, at the end of the discussion, this manager didn't give a rat's tail about the Mission of this company, or the Mission statement.

Hello, Mr. CEO. I'm sorry for boring you to tears. I'm almost done. Do you recall an email you sent to everyone in the company outlining all of the great reasons to stay there longer? One of those items was a statement about additional vacation time for those with more years. Prior to my departure, I gave a two-week notice. I explained to my manager part of the reason I struggled with the decision to leave, was because I'd be giving up four weeks a year of vacation. I was within months of it happening. My manager responded by saying: "That's no big deal."

That's no big deal. There you have it, Mr. CEO. That's no big deal. Once again, somebody made a liar out of you. The next time you send a company email enticing others to stay longer and you decide to make a list of those reasons, you can let that one off the list. You can also let the one about better advancement for those with more years off the list.

Here's another interesting fact. I mentioned I stayed an additional week to complete a huge upgrade for this company. Is it on my record at HR? No. Was I paid for my work that week? No, I was not. This is a biggie. I'll tell you why. My termination date (my last day of being a paid employee) had already passed. During the last week I was there, I was being paid by this company for vacation hours which I had accrued. So, I was technically on vacation. During my "Vacation" I was working for your company, and I was not technically an employee because my termination date was prior to my vacation. So, was this against company policy? Was this against state labor laws? If so, shouldn't my manager have been aware of this company policy or the state labor laws? Again, I'll repeat what I said before: "IT Management does what they want, when they want, if they want, how they want, and for who they want."

Where were you, Mr. CEO? I don't recall two weeks going by where I didn't see you at least once in your office, or out and about. During my last three weeks there, I didn't see you one single time. Not once. Were you away on vacation for those three weeks? I was going to drop by to let you know the big news about the possibility of me hosting a seminar in Las Vegas, but you weren't around. I didn't feel this was proper to do via a phone call. Something this big needed to be told face-to-face. I was brimming with excitement to share this great news with you, but you were nowhere to be found. I guess it wasn't meant to be.

I thought maybe you were on vacation. If so, I thought it strange that you'd be on vacation for three weeks in a row, during the building project. I guess it could have been another one of those weird "coincidences" that seem to follow me around. I'm not sure why the clinical systems manager didn't tell you. I'm not sure why neither of the two administrative directors didn't tell you. I don't know if the VP knew, but I suspect she did. I can only suspect, I have no proof. There's also a good chance she didn't know because the three managers who knew played the famous "don't ask, don't tell" game. It doesn't matter because even if she did know, I don't think she would have told you. That's my personal opinion based on my experience. So, back to the question. Where were you for three weeks? Did you somehow get involved in something which kept you away from your office for three weeks? Think long and hard. I won't tell you what I suspect, I just wanted you to know that I suspect I know what happened. Say that one ten times fast.

I believe I'm owed almost One Hundred and Fifty Thousand dollars for the last five years I worked there. I also believe I'm owed another One Hundred and Fifty Thousand dollars working as an independent contractor for my last week there. Why so much for my last week? We paid an outside consulting firm Twenty-Five Hundred dollars an hour for a system migration/upgrade. The consultant was there for two or three weeks. There were dozens of firms specializing in this kind of work. The work I did was even more specialized. I believe I may have been one of only five or six people in the country who had the knowledge and experience to complete the task I completed. Therefore, my hourly rate should have been much higher, but I rounded it down to an even twenty-five percent higher. So, we're up to about Three Hundred Thousand I'm now owed. Who should I send the bill to? Do you realize had I sued you mental anguish and pain and suffering could have been lumped on top of those figures? Do you know how much money it could have amounted to? No, it wouldn't have been millions. Juries don't award that kind of money anymore, unless it's a class action. But, this could have been a class action, had I went public.

Multiple employees from this department had various forms and/or types of retribution taken against them for being honest on the Online Survey. The issues which weren't addressed, nor even mentioned or talked about, would have included or involved dozens of employees from other departments. This company could have incurred a major amount of losses, litigation, and exposure to the tune of somewhere between ten to twenty million dollars, maybe more. In my opinion, the employees I mentioned in this story should all receive a check for no less than a million dollars each. I wonder if your new so-called allies would cough up the dough? I doubt it.

I wonder if you realize, Mr. CEO, how much damage could have been done if I'd went public with this information ten years ago? I think a reward is in order. How about a million dollars? I think that would be a fair amount. What about pain and suffering and mental anguish? Sorry, but I can't and won't put a price on that. Neither you or your company would have enough money for it if I did. Excuse me for a moment, I need to speak with the readers. Hello everyone, are you laughing? Remember: This is supposed to be a comedy.

What will you do now, Mr. CEO? How will you move forward? Will your life be different knowing when you look some of these managers in the eye, you're looking at bold-face liars, manipulators, conspirators, and violators of labor laws? Will you believe it was I who tipped off the Board of Directors about the plaza scam? Will you believe if it wasn't for me you might not be CEO? Or, you might have inherited a company with a huge boat anchor wrapped around it's neck? It doesn't really matter to me what you choose to believe at this time. I just wanted you to know the truth. I also wanted you to know your so-called "Pillars" statements were all bull-squat in the IT Department. The only thing those pillars were used for where I worked was to beat me into submission. Now, it is me doing the beating. I've got my own "Pillar" and I have "Faith" someone in this world will agree 100% with some of this report.

I've read about a subject known as "Workplace Bullying." I think I've just showed multiple examples of it taking place. The internet has a very good description and definition of workplace bullying. Nearly everything in one of those descriptions happened to me and it was all based on retaliation, which is against state labor laws. I was retaliated against because I was honest on the Online Survey.

Violence in the workplace. There's a good one. I'm grateful I'm not a violent person by nature. If I were, this story would have a different ending. If there was a violent ending, the shame of it is nobody would have ever known what caused it. Nobody would have ever known the truth. I thank God I'm not a violent person. And God helped me to show you the pen really is mightier than the sword. But, what about someone else? Could there be a person out there who was also shafted by this company? There is. I've already shown you there is. Could there be a person out there who might have violent tendencies or might suddenly "snap" after all these years and decide violence is the way to resolve it? I surely hope not. Maybe somebody will decide to be proactive and eliminate or reduce the risk of it happening. How would you do that? I'll keep my opinion to myself. I'm sure with all of the four-year degrees and vast amounts of knowledge now linked with this company someone will be smart enough to figure it out.

Some might feel since it's been about ten years ago they have nothing to worry about. Only time will tell. I believe you should be concerned. I believe in erring on the side of caution. Don't worry. If anything violent were to happen, I won't say I told you so. This story says it all. I'll tell you who might say "I told you so." Anyone who reads this book, sees the movie, or was also a victim of similar treatment by your company, might say: "He told you so," or "I'm not surprised."

Chapter 20

As shared earlier, there was never a direct impact to patient care concerning these issues. What about indirect impact? Here are some examples of the indirect impact it has on patient care.

Hospitals receive most of their revenues from the insurance companies and from the government. When idiotic things go on where common sense isn't being applied or used, the cost of this lunacy comes out of your pocket. You pay an insurance company for coverage. You visit a hospital and the insurance company pays the bill. Is anyone concerned some of these funds were wasted on a committee to decide what kind of coffee the IT Department was going to start buying and using?

Employee retention. How much overhead is there in the HR Department and Marketing relating to new employee recruitment? When employees leave due to poor management tactics, it's costing more in the long run than properly addressing the real problem. And these costs come out of funds paid to this company by the insurance companies and the government. I don't think any of these funds came from charitable contributions. Maybe they came from a budgeted line-item amount known as The Idiot Fund.

What will happen now? Will this company take out the trash or will their new "Allies" give them a nudge in that direction? Will they simply not comment about it? Maybe they'll start a campaign to discredit me. That wouldn't surprise me. It wouldn't surprise me if they were to fabricate information and slander me in order to discredit me. I don't care what they do. I suspect they might even try to come up with some plausible, idiotic explanation for these things happening. Maybe they'll do as the Pharaoh did with Moses. Maybe the Pharaoh (or the CEO) will say: "Let him rant that people will know him to be totally crazy." Crazy he is, but dishonest he isn't. I have a question for these so-called new allies: After reading this, would you hire any one of these managers to work for you? If the answer is no, then they shouldn't be working for you now. If the answer is yes, then your company is another example of what's wrong with a lot of companies in this country.

I read something about how your company now claims to value your employees feedback, or opinions, or something along those lines. I don't believe it. No way. No how. I know how the game is played. I bet it's played the same way it was played when I worked there. If an idea can save money or make money but involves stepping on somebody's toes that are high up on the political or financial ladder, it's not gonna happen. If an idea would create common-sense efficiency, but would require others (again on the political or financial ladder) to be held to certain standards of accountability, it's not gonna happen. I say this because a majority of the managers who were involved in everything I've shared about in this book are still working there. And I truly believe they are probably still doing: What they want, when they want, if they want, how they want and for who they want.

I want you to know, Mr. CEO, I now have something very special to me. It's not a Super Bowl ring, nor is it an Olympic Gold medal. It's not the trophy for winning the Daytona 500. It's not a piece of paper hanging on my wall as a reminder. It's not a piece of paper that will be hidden behind a closed door during the holiday season, if you and the head of the board come by for a visit. It's simply the knowledge that: I was the first to accomplish great things at a company I once worked for. I was once the best, or one of the best, in this country at something, maybe one of the best in the world, but nobody cared. I know it and God knows it. God knows everything and God knows the truth. My future and my destiny are in God's hands.

If anyone chooses to speak about this book in public or the media, don't refer to me as a disgruntled employee. As I said before: It begins with dis, but the word is discrimination. By the CEO's very own words, I was discriminated against. There's information on record at HR which proves I was discriminated against. It's factual information and HR has it. You just need to know what to look for and how to find it. In closing, I would like to share a little poem with you concerning the future.

I'm writing a screenplay with tales galore

It surely will open some huge cans of worms

Some won't believe the things I'll report

This story is just the tip of the iceberg

More of the story is gonna come out

And some are gonna panic

Because it wasn't the tip of the iceberg

That sunk the Titanic

How about a movie for your video shelf?

If I can't get Tarantino, I'll produce it myself

And I'll wear a new hat in the director's chair

Lights camera action: Now I'm the puppeteer

I'm hoping a movie deal will be inked

But a mini-series would also make my day

A closing note from the Author:

I welcome the opportunity to speak with anyone who would like to talk about this story. I also welcome input from anyone who has also had a bad experience involving this company. This story can be changed and updated at any time. This story can also have more added to it. You can Contact me via Facebook.com/merlinwaltzauthor

I would like to thank you for reading my story. I hope you learned something from it.

Hoping that our paths cross again –

Merlin

Other Books Currently Available:

The Catcher

Grudge Money

Two Twins One Gun

Stored Shorts – A collection of short stories

Poetry On Parade – A small collection of Poetry